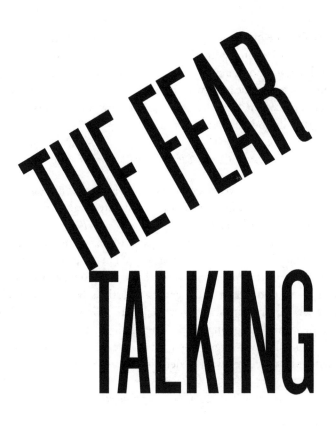

THE FEAR TALKING

Anxiety is the most common form of mental distress and of course overlaps with normal human emotion. Yet it can be overwhelming and disabling and a gateway to other mental ill health notably depression and self-medication with alcohol and other substances. This engaging account throws a spotlight on how anxiety impacts on everyday life and relationships.

– Patrick McGorry,
Professor of Youth Mental Health, University of Melbourne

As a nurse of many years' experience I have heard countless stories of human distress and learned how to hold myself apart from other people's suffering. Chris Westoby's *The Fear Talking* expertly but gently slips past my professional guard to engage me in the life of a young man suffering from anxiety. The story is interesting, humorous, distressing, compassionate and intriguing, and as I read, I begin to understand the mental contortions behind the social paralysis anxiety brings, and then to discern its impact on self, family, friendships, schooling, work – the whole of life. Read this book, and you will never forget it. As a narrative it's fascinating. As the memoir of a life lived with anxiety, it's incomparable.

– Peter Draper,
Emeritus Professor of Nursing Education, University of Hull

In *The Fear Talking*, Chris Westoby achieves the well-nigh impossible, giving us a fully immersive account of adolescent anxiety, allowing the reader to feel and experience with the narrator. If one of the main aims of the memoir form is to induce empathy in readers, Westoby's memoir succeeds brilliantly. The reader comes away with a new and profound understanding of what mental illness feels like from within.

– Jonathan Taylor,
Associate Professor Creative Writing, University of Leicester

Chris Westoby shows us what it is to make use of the resonant power of words to offer a portal into what it is really like. A vital touchstone for public and health professionals alike, to understand deeply, to see and to learn from first person experience.

– Kathleen T. Galvin,
Professor of Nursing Practice, University of Brighton

This book offers young people an insight into the range of unique ways the world can be experienced and the chance to reflect on their own struggles and know they are not alone in these. It offers health care practitioners a first-hand and powerful opportunity to understand how it feels to live with anxiety as a young person. The book has been used as a tool for those educating student practitioners in the field of mental health to support development of empathy and an enhanced emotional vocabulary. I have recommended this book to my academic colleagues, my students and my children.

– Dr Judith Dyson,
Reader Healthcare Research, Birmingham City University

The Fear Talking offers educators in the caring professions something which can generate feelings, opening up the space for students, professionals, trainees to talk about not only the lived experience of others but to engage with what they themselves feel. At once shocking and relatable, the immersive literary style coupled with the real-world experience acts as a means to foster empathy and reflection in the reader at a deeper level than traditional case studies. *The Fear Talking* offers us access to not only the story of a life marked by anxiety, although it tells that story so engagingly. It creates a feeling of anxiety in the reader, but with a sensibility of care and a common humanity. Chris Westoby cares for his readers and allows them to explore his experience and their own experience of being affected by that experience in a safe space. In doing so, he models a sensibility of care for readers to consider and discuss. My students have benefited from engaging with this work in their ability to make sense of experience and to challenge assumptions.

– Dr Timothy Buescher,
Programme Director for Mental Health Nursing, University of Hull

CHRIS WESTOBY

THE FEAR TALKING

THE TRUE
STORY OF A
YOUNG MAN
AND ANXIETY

BARB
ICAN
PRESS

First published in Great Britain by Barbican Press in 2020

Registered office: 1 Ashenden Road, London E5 0DP

www.barbicanpress.com

@barbicanpress1

Cover by Jason Anscomb

A CIP catalogue for this book is available from the British Library

ISBN: 978-1-909954-44-1

Typeset in Adobe Garamond

Typeset in India by Imprint Digital Ltd

About the Author

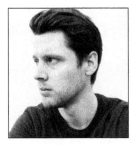

This is a true story. You'll learn a lot about Chris and the life-long anxiety he fought to keep secret.

Born and raised in Barton, on the Lincolnshire side of the Humber, a bus took him to college in Scunthorpe. He earned money on a paper round and making windows. But leaving home triggered unceasing visions of shame, distress, illness. It became unbearable to go anywhere, and impossible to explain why. He has written the book he wishes he could've read back then, to help understand what was happening and know he wasn't alone.

He hopes it might get into the hands of others who need it.

Chris Westoby obtained his Creative Writing PhD at the University of Hull, where he is now Programme Director of the Hull Online Creative Writing MA. He lectures in Creative Writing, guest lectures in subjects of mental health, teaches reflective writing to Mental Health Nursing students, and runs cross-faculty writing workshops. He works in research, collecting the stories of others.

He still makes windows.

The sequels are being lived; they're being written. His condition is a never-ending story.

Twitter @ChrisWestoby / @feartalking
Instagram westo90 / feartalking

Mum & Dad

Orlando

There's a massive *crack* in the sky and some of the bystanders shriek. The space shuttle *Discovery* appears through the highest clouds; the last echoes of its sonic boom roll around the lake.

Another vicious, hot day. It's summer 2006 and we're in Florida, stood in a layby near the outskirts of Kennedy Space Center. My family and me. Our Grand Voyager's tyres are powdered white by the chalky ground, its doors wide open to stop the heat building inside.

Other groups are staggered about, all beside their cars, all looking up. They chat happily now and raise their cameras. What a picture. A *shuttle* coming down from *space*, over the busy carriageway, above the pristine lake. Right before our eyes. And I've heard this might be the end of the last mission it ever takes. That's pretty damn cool, surely. But I can't focus.

My left hand holds the empty Coke beaker I've carried around since our first morning here, when we waited for that downpour to stop before a big stunt show and I thought I was going to be sick. The idea is: if I'm ill, maybe I can, like, put my mouth in this beaker and look as though I'm drinking and people won't know I'm throwing up. At least it won't go on the floor.

Unless the vomit fills the beaker up and it overflows.

I should carry two.

My right hand taps the little pocket on the hip of my shorts. Two bumps under the cotton. Yes, the Imodium tablets are still in there.

That's what matters.

Beaker and tablets. They're with me. It'll be alright.

I've counted every minute of the drive from the apartment to this layby, watched the speed limits of different roads and whether Dad obeys them, how long we've idled at each red light, how busy the roads are and whether that's slowed us down. Because every minute we travel means the journey back is another minute longer.

God, we're miles away.

I'm sweating, swallowing into a dry throat.

'You getting a picture, Chris?' Mum twists round to me, shielding her eyes from the sun.

'It's too far away.'

We watch *Discovery* come all the way down to the tree line across the lake, and I wonder if that's its nose still glowing or glare from the sun. A woman in salmon shorts and black shoes starts to clap, then lowers her hands when no one joins her.

My head rests in my hands as our people-carrier enters traffic again. Kennedy Space Center is meant to be an hour and a half from our apartment in Lake Buena Vista, but it's been longer than that. I knew it would be. Dad either underestimates or lies when it comes to journey times.

In the Center's garden of old rockets, shuttles and satellites, I squint up at a marble wall with names chipped into it, shuffle after my family, up some steps and into a decommissioned shuttle with tin foil for wallpaper.

Behind her back, Mum squeezes one hand inside the other. Her mouth is nipped closed. It's me she's pissed off with.

We file into a theatre and join the small crowd finding their seats in the dark. A short film about the heroism of space travel plays, with CGI aerial shots of the moon and astronauts who bounce along in slow motion.

An invisible door opens beside the screen and a portly man steps in from the sunlight. Whilst talking to the audience he tips forward on his toes, backwards on his heels, and gently smacks his closed fist into his palm. He explains the **day ahead of us**, that there are **three** parts to the tour on different parts of the massive grounds, and a **bus** will take us from area to area.

Fuck me, I thought this was it. I thought we'd seen and done Kennedy already and were heading back soon.

I pick at the edge of my beaker and follow the group outside to queue for a bus. We're shepherded into a maze of railings, which from above must look like a diagram of small intestines – doubling back again and again. Big metal fans blow down on us and make no difference. I study the tour leaflet and try to draw comfort that once we're in Area 2 there's an optional bus that runs straight back to the reception. Pat my pocket. Tablets are there. Try to swallow, feeling really sick. I think I'm getting something. I'm so hot.

Of course you're hot – it's Florida.

No, it's like I'm getting sick.

Everything's sticky. The floor sucks at my feet.

I can't just make us leave. There are five of us; it would take too long to convince them all. They'll say I'm being stupid. And I can't drive the rent-a-car or run away. I'm not free. Even if I get us to go, my family can see me all that way home in the car. Close enough to knock knees, to smell each other's breath. I can't vanish.

Our bus stops in the middle of the concrete expanse between Area 1 and 2.

The bus has stopped.

Panic, like cold water, trickles under the skin of my chest, down my limbs.

Maybe our halt is part of the routine and we'll be moving again soon. It must be part of the tour. Nothing's wrong. Surely we're about to set off again.

To stay busy, I calculate the travel times from one Area station to the next, using my fingers as rulers on the little pamphlet map. I estimate the travel time from here, back to the entrance, to the car, down the 528 to the apartment. My palm sweat dampens the pamphlet; flecks of blue and white print stick to my skin.

Is there somewhere to hide out there? Foliage to take cover in or walls to climb over? It's a baking emptiness.

We're still not moving.

Have we broken down?

The driver announces that the *Discovery* shuttle is being taxied past us.

'This is an amazing lucky chance,' she says. 'We'll be sitting tight for about twenny, twenny-five minutes. But please remain in your seats.'

Forty-odd people jump up and fight for a view out the right-hand side where I'm sat, cramming into each other, cresting over me.

The gigantic shuttle comes along, surrounded by machines that flash amber lights. A convoy of black cars and SUVs follow. Officials walk either side of the congregation.

'Please, sit *down*!' our driver says.

I am!

I rest an elbow on either thigh, fingers pinching the plastic cup, head hanging off my shoulders, ready to be sick. The herd of tourists around me dissolves into a rush of images behind my eyes.[1]

'Is anyone getting a picture? Chris?' Mum says.

My older brother James takes the camera and snaps *Discovery's* crawling approach. The shuttle and its convoy are barely twenty metres from us before it turns towards a hidden part of the complex.

Our bus driver, sick of our shit, wastes no time getting us to Area 2.

'I think I need to go back. I reckon I'm gonna be sick,' I say aside to Mum under a grid shadow on the concrete, opening the half-disintegrated map. 'There's a bus that goes straight from here back to the entrance, look.'

'For God's sake. We've come all this way, Chris. You're completely ruining it. Moping round and saying you're sick. "Woe is me." The whole trip, you've done nothing but sulk. If you didn't want to come today, you should've stayed at the bloody apartment.'

I *wanted* to stay at the apartment. I pleaded but they wouldn't go without me. I'm not sulking; I'm sick. I don't want to ruin their holiday. Just hide me.

She digs some paracetamols from her purse and tells me to take a couple.

'I'm not in pain.'

---

[1] I picture the vomit falling out my mouth: a quiet descends on the bus; passengers retreat away from me like I'm a live grenade; their remarks of disgust spread through the crowd with the smell. Do I hear laughter? Sympathy? Word reaches the front. The driver announces over the tannoy that, 'We'll get cleaned up at the next station.' Vomit down my front. My t-shirt, shorts and boxers stick to me. Vomit down my legs, in my shoes. We get back to the car and Mum puts a towel over the seat before I sit down. All the windows are rolled down for two hours. Maybe I'm sick again.

'It can take the edge off,' she says.

That doesn't make sense but fuck it. I pop them from their foil and swallow them down. And despite knowing she's desperately throwing placebos at me, it works.

By the time we're heading to Area 3, I'm fine. Fine! Does it matter whether it's in my head? Paracetamol just thins the blood, my chemistry-proficient friend once told me. Maybe my blood is too thick, that's why I always feel sick. And this is actually helping.

I take dozens of pictures throughout the rest of the day: my younger brother Jordan standing under the disassembled rocket, the moon buggy, a turtle that floats up from the murk of a pond to snap at a bug caught in the thick surface tension.

We drive into a storm. The streetlights wake and Dad has the wipers on full chat. I spot the three steel hotel tower skeletons and know we're about to arrive at the resort. A short dash from the car to our apartment block soaks us through. Puddles have formed on the turquoise floor of the open corridors. James unlocks the apartment door and icy air conditioning touches my wet skin.

I've made it.

Mum goes into her bedroom and shuts the door.

Behind the counter, Dad pats a new filter into the coffee machine and Jordan takes a slimy donut from the box. Me and James sit on the wicker sofa, flicking through today's photos on the camera screen. I was behind the lens in most, but in the few where you see me, I look perfectly calm – cocky, even – both before and after the moment the paracetamols took effect. You'd never guess what it was really like.

* * *

Swampy woods go by on our way to more theme parks. I follow my family around as though on a lead, take pictures, wait whilst they queue for rides. Daydream about going home. In strange moments, like waking up mid-sleepwalk, I find myself stroking the soft feathers of an exotic bird, ploughing into the splash pool at the bottom of a massive water slide, tasting a tart raspberry smoothie and crunching the blended ice. A screen is lifted, and the world is loud and sharp.

In the evenings, any plans my parents make for the following day torment me until I fall asleep. In the mornings, I wake hoping they might have forgotten, and try to suggest we hang out by the pool.

One night, when the lights are off, I recall that scene in *Return of the King*: Sam has the half-dead Frodo in his arms, whose spirits he attempts to rekindle by reciting the quaint details of their home. I imagine that longing West Country voice listing off the arrangement of my own bedroom in England. Even in the privacy of my head, the thought embarrasses me. Sixteen years old, and I can't be abroad for a fortnight without being homesick.

But then, is it homesickness? Home isn't what I'm pining for. Just a way out of this nightmare, that's all.

Over and over, I work out the days left until we go home. Count, count, add, subtract. To the hour of departure, hour of landing in Manchester, hour of arrival in Barton. But Mum and Dad have worked themselves to the bone for this holiday. They must see me having fun.

Don't ruin it.

We get as far as the dock and join the queues for a ferry. Above the tourists' heads I see the black moat and Magic Kingdom's iconic castle lit up in neon pinks and purples.

One boat recedes to the far shore and another approaches us, unzipping the island's reflection. Having to take a boat to this supposed place of dreams to watch the fireworks – it's all I've thought about today. And the panic that threatened to peak as we arrived in the car park tonight now boils over.

'I need to go back,' I say to Mum, hoping James and Jordan don't hear me. 'I need to leave.'

Anger lowers her eyebrows, but she doesn't refuse outright like at Kennedy.

'What's going on?' Dad says.

'Chris wants to leave.'

'Oh, right. What's wrong?'

'I don't feel good,' I say.

'Right.' Dad looks at the ferry, now halting by the dock and opening its little gate to let the people from Magic Kingdom get off. Our queue starts filing on. 'We'd better go then.'

'What's happening?' James says.

'We're off. Chris doesn't feel well,' says Dad.

'What's wrong?' Jordan asks me.

I don't answer and march to the shuttle that takes us back to the car, hoping my family will follow suit. The prickling sickness builds in me and I'm petrified I'll shit myself. On the shuttle, warm air flaps my hair and the man on the intercom hopes we've had a magical day. We get off and walk to the car. My family move so fucking slow. We should be sprinting.

The car's musty, foreign smell fills my head. Its acceleration lurches my insides. I put my head in my hands and send my desperate prayer.

Dear God, please help me. Don't let me be ill right now. Even if I have to be massively sick when we get back to the flat, just let it be then. Please. Just not now. Not now. I'm begging. I know there's a time someone has to ask for help and they get, like, one wish. If this is my one wish, I'm spending it. Let me get back before I'm sick. I won't ask for this again.

It's a while before I dare look up from my hands and recognise the streetlights that file by above me, their glow panning through the car.

Thank you, thank you, thank you.

Part 1

1

In my dreams I'm still there, swirling through the undercurrent. I wake up and see the blinds in my bedroom, the neighbour's security light shining through, casting pale stripes on the wall, and remember I'm home. It's September, and this is England.

The Humber is a broad, silt and shit-stained estuary yawning into the North Sea, and Barton grows on its southern bank. You know you're nearly here when you see the Humber Bridge's towers on the horizon, looking over us. I've never lived anywhere else. Nor really gone anywhere else, unless my parents drive me. Since one brave trip to see *Pirates of the Caribbean* three years ago, I've avoided buses entirely, and made countless wincing excuses why I can't join my friends when they travel outside of Barton.

That's got to change now. School's behind us and John Leggott in Scunthorpe is the closest college. It's barely twenty miles away, but the bus route sticks to the back roads and threads through every village. An hour's ride, twice a day. I think about it all the time, whether the bus might be too much for me, but compared to America this should be nothing. And think about the big Tesco a couple of miles from Leggott: surely, if it comes to it, I can walk there. I'll hide in a toilet cubicle until Mum or Dad picks me up. If they can leave work. There's all the tablets I keep in the side pocket of my bag. And I've downloaded a few episodes of *Scrubs* onto my iPod, in case things get so bad that I need a happy distraction. Things are fine. Well, maybe.

Stepping aboard on the first cool morning wakes the nerves, when the doors close behind me and the next stop isn't until Ferriby. Not that getting off there would do me any good.

Nearly everyone in our friendship group from school got a pass for the main bus, the 350. But me, Boris, George, Emma and Sebastian are on the decrepit double-decker 360, which teems like an ant nest with people we don't know. Down the aisle, up the stairs, down the upstairs aisle, we're packed in until the driver's forced to plough straight past the village bus stops and give the outraged folk waiting there a wide-armed shrug.

There's a slight weakness in my legs as we arrive at Leggott. Home feels *really* far away. If not by distance then accessibility, what it'd take to get back, like a drawbridge has risen between us. My fingertips find the bumps in the mini pocket of my jeans and just touch them for a second.

Two Imodium tablets. Here for me.

We cross the main road at lunchtime to lie on one of the sport fields. I pinch the crispy, cut grass from the alive grass, roll it into an owl pellet ball and throw it at Boris, who catches it in his mouth. Little wisps of smoke rise from the knots of students lying about in the warmth. Boys get up to play footy. A Nerf ball arcs over us, between two parties taking it in turns to throw. A guy runs around his friends with a screaming girl over his shoulder, who reaches down to fish for his pants and yanks them halfway up his back. A queue forms in front of an ice cream truck that's mounted the kerb and parked on the grass. There are thousands here, all my age. I've heard that some people get frightened by the crowds.

Emma puts make-up on next to me as we clatter past Scunthorpe's foreign shops.

'She's off to see Tommy. And she really can't be bothered,' George says, who's turned round from the seat in front, her arm draped over the back.

'Why not? What's wrong with him?' I say.

'Dumping him,' George mouths.

Emma's got a spot just below the tip of her nose. She brings a tissue to her face as though to sneeze, but I know what she's really doing, and I pretend to look forward. When she brings the tissue down the spot's deflated and nearly invisible. She holds up a pocket mirror to check. A little drop of honey-coloured liquid collects where the spot was and jiggles with the movement of the bus until she wipes it again.

George turns back round and talks to Boris about transferring to the 350. Boris starts singing 'In The Morning' by The Coral, which makes me picture the song's stop-motion music video and feel uncomfortable.

Me and Emma flick through the erotic book she's reading and point out funny lines in a chapter where the main character gets fucked against an underground statue.

Emma reminisces about school, despite us only leaving three months ago.

'You always avoided me,' she says in her London accent, joking but with an "admit it!" kind of tone.

'I wasn't avoiding you.'

'You did. Just because you were the popular boy at school—'

'No way.'

'—with all the popular girlfriends.'

'No way.'

'With the Corner Crew. Hanging out with Sophia and all them lot. I was at The Wall. Like, the *lesser* place.'

'Me, Ryan and Ben *started* The Corner, matter of fact.'

'Oh yeah?'

'We just liked pissing about on those yellow bars. We didn't know half the year group would end up there. You could've come. It wasn't members-only. In fact, you *did* hang out with us last year.'

'Only because I'm with Tommy and sort of tagged along. You never spoke to me anyway.'

'Because you're a nobody.'

Emma gasps and prods my ribs, repeating it back half a dozen times in answer to nearly everything I say for the next half hour.

'Oh, because I'm a nobody!'

Her giggle's really shrill; sometimes she just can't stop laughing. She goes on about being "hypo". A lot of my friends think she's annoying.

As we pick up speed towards Ferriby, she puts a leg over mine. I can't decide whether I like it.

Literature, Language, Media and Fine Art are the butt of smirking jokes for Ryan and Ben, both high-scoring scientists, but that's what I study.

Twice a week, I even get to go home early. The bus from college to Barton only runs at the start and end of the day, so on the first "early day", me and Ben walk into Scunthorpe's town centre to catch one from the station. We rifle through the albums in HMV, grab some cheap Arabian Coke from Home Bargains, and wait for the "Paragon Hull" bus that takes us through Roxby, Winterton, Winteringham and Ferriby. All the windows are open and warm air billows through the carriage. Ben's on the seat facing me. His eyes are closed, his earphones in. I know he's listening to Radiohead, like me. The wind makes his gigantic afro-like hair lash about.

* * *

My uncle Harvey gets in touch: he's fitting replacement windows near college and asks if I want to help out in the afternoons I don't have lessons. Two hundred metres *further* than college. But the house he's working at is slightly closer to the big Tesco. And I could use the money. My weekly paper round – fast becoming something to be ashamed of – fetches less than it used to. I head out Leggott's main gate, past the tennis courts and footy fields, down a steep hill to find the house Harvey's van is parked in front of. Dead leaves float out from the woods beside me; the path's carpeted with them, all flattened down to mush, giving off the sweet autumnal smell of rot.

Harvey spends the afternoon sawing through a massive roll of tissue paper, and I can't figure why this is necessary.

He drives me back in the van, through the lowlands of the Ancholme Valley's shallow slopes.

Harvey's a middle-aged bachelor living with my grandparents, with a perfect egg-shaped bald patch atop his thick hair. Shouldered from one family business he co-created and failing to make it with the second one he started alone, Harvey gets work where he can. He can drive with his knee (so there's something going for him), his packed lunch on his lap, his hands free to peel three tangerines.

The nights are pulling in.

We stop at a bungalow in the middle of nowhere and a blinding security light comes on. A woman in pyjamas comes into the spotlight on the brick drive. She trades flirty insults with my uncle as we unload scrap wood from our job into her garage. Harvey has an arrangement with her, so he says once we're back on the road: he brings her scrap wood, and something is given in return. Whatever that means.

I think about how much wood was already in her garage.

The trees that flitter by in the dark: not ideal, but an effective place to hide. I could make my uncle pull over, jump out whilst the van's moving if I have to, hop this low wall – careful of the bramble growing over it – and keep running. Maybe crouch down in the undergrowth. Or even lie on my side and put up with the bed of wet leaves soaking into my clothes. Would Harvey understand well enough to leave me there?

Probably not.

But it's an emergency plan I've mentally rehearsed all day. And all yesterday. Now we're nearly home, a safe fifteen minutes to go, it seems so stupid: worrying that I was off to fit windows.

I shake my head.

Worried that I was off to fit windows!

'You want a tangie?' my uncle says. The pack-up box balances on his lap; it tilts like a boat as he steers with his knees whilst his hands peel away at the fruit.

We stop for the railway crossing and I feel sleepy.

The smell of citrus rind splitting from the flesh mixes with the van's heaters.

Amber lights glow behind the dashboard dials.

Static frays a quiet voice on the half tuned-in radio.

'Nah, thanks,' I say.

2

I take paracetamol before breakfast to keep a sickness away. The next dose is on my way to Language, as I cross the courtyard lawns and keep a distance from some batty kid who launches a juggling diabolo higher than the science block. His eyes scrunch in the sunlight as he watches it fly and his gum-chewing pauses until it lands back on the string with a cheer from his mates. Outside the mobile classrooms, a guy's having a fit on the path; his friend has put a coat under his jerking head and now sits cross-legged nearby reading a book. 'It's alright, he's fine,' she says. I remember the third paracetamol dose halfway through the final lesson. By now the sickness has hollowed.

Boris finds me and we leave through the main entrance. The low sun's in our eyes. Leggott's towering headmaster stands on the paving that leads down to the gates and the queue of rumbling buses beyond. He's waving and says bye to people as they go past like he knows them all.

'Bye, Chris!' he says to me when I catch his eyes.

'See you,' I say, then snap round to Boris and murmur, 'How the fuck does he know my name?'

We climb the hill to Glover Road, where our lowly 360 waits. 'Have you heard about Maccy D's getting shut down?' Boris says. 'Fucking jizz burgers. A guy was spaffing in all the burgers. And he had herpes. Some girl caught it and they traced it back or some bollocks. I'm not really sure. It might not be true.'

'So it was someone who was making the burgers that jizzed in them?'

'Yeah.'

'Which Maccy's?'

'The one near big Tescos.'

'How didn't anyone notice him wanking into the burgers? Did he cook them and arrange all the lettuce and sauce with one hand, with his dick in the other hand wanking away? Or did he just sneak round the pre-made Big Macs and, you know, slip each one a quick *whoop?*' The more I act out the McDonald's man, the more Boris is laughing.

'I don't know!' he shouts, getting worked up. 'He just had a little jar and smeared a tiny bit on each one, maybe. Not enough to notice. He just went *shhhh*—' Boris strokes a finger down my cheek '—on each bap, and left his seed.'

'And his herpes.'

Emma and George emerge from the snicket.

'Oh hello,' George says. 'Where'd you come from?'

'Walked round front.'

'David Linell knew Chris's name,' Boris says.

'He's got an eidetic memory,' Emma says.

'"Ee's got an eeditic mimury",' Boris squeaks and kicks Emma in the leg.

'Fuck's sake, Boris. Piss off.' She brushes dusty mud off her thigh.

Boris gets out his pebble-shaped MP3 player, puts one earphone in and sings along to Christina Aguilera.

Chavs from Lindsey are sat at the back of the top deck, throwing abuse and exercise books at everyone in front. The girls pass make-up discs to the boys, who hurl them like skimming stones down the carriage, bursting into dust on the backs of the heads that try to keep their eyes forward and ignore it all. Someone withdraws to tell the driver. I gather shards of the make-up from the floor and throw them back. George starts giving the chavs a weird telling off that makes me feel like a wuss.

When it's my stop I go down and say to the driver, 'Thanks for sorting that lot upstairs out for us. That felt like a really safe journey.'

'What am I supposed to do? Throw them off?' he shouts, arms tensed above that big steering wheel, fingers splayed.

'Yes!' I say from the pavement.

He twats a button and the doors close.

'You're probably kicked off the bus now,' a stranger says beside me.

'Maybe.'

The bus disappears down Ferriby road, George still upstairs.

I hope she finds out what I said to the driver.

3

The sickness doesn't go. It's the first feeling I'm aware of when I wake up: an invisible thumb gently pressing the base of my throat. I imagine what concoction swills around in my stomach as I walk from lesson to lesson, or stagnates like a swamp as I sit still in class and try to think of anything else, even when my stomach is empty, which is most mornings. I avoid the concrete steps in the courtyard that juggle my insides. And if stairs can't be avoided, I keep my climb smooth and slow. The bumpy roads and the bus's deep idle rattle shake it all up. But then I get home, go to the gym, and the feeling's gone.

Paracetamol's a must. Four-hour intervals, every day. I keep stocked up at the Spar we walk to at the end of college's road.

Getting on the bus is harder. The journey length plays on my mind. Its unstoppable route. To step on board is to commit myself to an hour rammed in tight between passengers without hiding places if I get ill. I could barely squeeze myself through the throng to the entrance if I needed to jump off, let alone convince the driver to pull over unless there's a stop. And if there's a stop, the people hanging around it will see me.

And what if it's that driver I upset? Why would *he* let me off if I asked?

The destination is hardly better: two thousand students I should be composed in front of, not a puking mess. Many have camera phones that could take a picture of me. A picture to pass around. To spread. Classrooms are silent with a neutral smell: a blank canvas that any sickness episode would soil.

Maybe it's because of the wireless routers they've got here. People complain that the signals give them headaches. Why not nausea too?

The clammy Media Studies classroom at the top of all those stairs – it's always dark and close. The windows are locked behind glowing blinds. Computer towers, desperate to cool down, suck in hot air and radiate hotter air. Whenever someone speaks, their voice seems to come from right by my ear. The air is thick, like trying to inhale aspic; it clogs behind my eyes. I can taste it: the room, maybe, the people, the situation, being up here.

Lunch ends on an October afternoon. We're sat around one of the circular tables in the Maggy May, Leggott's huge canteen that tries to be a club with its purple walls, chrome railings lining the upper floor and big speakers at the mercy of student DJs. Now it's getting cold outside, we spend nearly all our free periods in here.

Our round of Bullshit is cut short; my friends chuck their cards down and depart to their different lessons, but I don't move.

The thought of that Media classroom, where I'm meant to be heading now – I can't do it. I feel sick.

And if I'm too sick to go to Media, I can't go into town to get a bus home either.

I'm stranded.

My eyes start darting around all the faces in here.

'Have you got a free, Chris?' Webster asks, noticing I haven't got up.

'Yeah,' I lie.

'We're off home. There's a seat left, if you want a lift back,' he offers, pointing over his shoulder with his car keys.

I'll escape, just this once.

Five of us pile into Webster's 90s Golf. He takes the winding Pheasant Way, then turns onto Racer's Lane and rags his Golf until it's juddering at a hundred and ten miles per hour. I'm in the middle back seat with a limp belt over my waist. We go up a hump in the road and as it crests we float from our seats for a moment and my bladder tingles. We overtake a Honda. Scale another blind hump. A crawling tractor appears right in our face and an oncoming car blocks us from overtaking it. Webster mashes the brakes, cuts into a tiny pull-in and the car goes *bang* over the stones and the back end swerves away. The tyres find grip and we bump back onto the road, ahead of the tractor. The Golf wiggles back into a straight line.

A moment passes and Webster goes, 'Ha ha ha ha.' He turns round to us all. 'Fuck *that*.'

That would've killed us, just then, if that pull-in wasn't in that exact place.

'Nice,' I say, and hope this rescue might happen again. What would I have done without it?

But by the weekend, Webster writes his car off in a crash.

4

'It's just another day in the office for him, Christopher.'

'What do I say?' I laugh and put my head on my crossed arms at the kitchen table.

'You don't need a script. He'll just say, "Now, Mr. Westoby, what seems to be the problem?" and away you go.' Mum pushes in the dishwasher tray, shuts its door and hits "go". She throws the dish sponge in front of me. 'You can give the table a wipe whilst you're sitting there looking pretty.'

'He'll just say I'm being stupid or it's in my head.' I wipe each placemat, stack them up and wipe the table.

'You're not going to know until you go see.'

The rotund doctor has a pepper beard and magnified eyes behind rectangular glasses. He gets me to lie on a thin leather bed with my shirt pulled up and my trousers undone. He presses on my stomach here and there with big cold fingers.

'Do you actually vomit?'

'So far, no. But it feels like I'm about to.'

'Any diarrhoea?'

'No, no.'

How does he say such a word so openly?

'Hmm. Okay.' He signals for me to button up and join him back at the desk.

I get a prescription for a drug called Stemetil.

As soon as the white package is handed over to me at the pharmacy I take one, and prepare to feel the queasiness lift. This could be it. I'm taken care of. Bring on tomorrow.

Over the next few weeks, I try to wean myself off paracetamol now I've got a proper replacement, but end up taking both. Stemetil doesn't do much. Is it even a real drug? Or was the doctor amusing me, thinking I'm some sad worrier? The tablets look like tea sweeteners – maybe that's all they are. Better to stay on them, in case, but let's bump up the paracetamol dosage and pop them every third hour. They take an hour to work, according to an advert I once saw, so really I'm just keeping on top of their slow activation, rather than having that hour of sour sickness between doses.

I take another afternoon off college. Then another. A full day is a believable length of time to potentially be caught out sick. The longer I stay, the higher the chances, so I itch and itch to leave. Early buses home are nearly empty most of the time: a couple of grannies or a young mother with two prams and six carrier bags. When in an afternoon lesson, I picture that crowded, standard-time bus home. I eat more mints, take more tablets, hope the nausea won't get worse.

You might argue college isn't off to a great start.

Has Florida fucked me up?

That night waiting for the ferry, the shuttle landing, the Caesar salads, slimy donuts, stepping on cracks, shuffling after my family, my mates in the tree before I left.

No, it can't be that.

I make myself get on the bus every morning, but need more and more paracetamol and Stemetil to take the edge off this constant sickness. Eating makes me want to hurl and certain foods *aren't right* so it's better to not eat at all.

5

It's early November. Emma's made sure to sit with me on the ride home. She laughs and laughs. It's dead easy and feels good. It doesn't matter if my own laughs are a bit forced. On some of the recent journeys, I've even put my arm around her.

Like tonight.

Yes there's George, who I fancied before, but she's shagging a twenty-five year-old sock salesman now, so when I hear Emma's got a thing for me, I think *why not?*

Beneath my feet I feel our bus drop into crawl gear for the last hill, where trees form a tunnel and even cyclists overtake us. It's nearly dark; the lights blink on inside, and all we can see through the windows are our own reflections.

Over the grinding engine, I say, 'So I've heard you like me.'

No reply at first – we were laughing at my impression of the Scissor Sisters only seconds ago – and then, 'I do. I thought you still liked George.'

'Not really.'

'Oh right,' she says. Under my arm, her little shoulders come up to her cheeks.

Timed just right as we come into Barton, I say, 'So shall we say we're together?'

'Yeah.'

I kiss her whilst pressing the bell to stop the bus. Grin and step off. As it pulls away again and my nose fills with tart exhaust fumes, I see her already texting me.

Later on, I'm out on my weekly paper round, dragging a massive fluorescent trolley of advert pages up the hills of my neighbourhood. My feet are already getting cold.

I can't have a girlfriend. There'll be things we have to do together, places we have to go. I'll text Emma tomorrow and say I made a cock-up and would rather not date. That I've been arrogant.

On my iPod, 'Rootless Tree' from Damien Rice's awkward second album plays. In the last stretch of the song I count him cry "let me out!" fifty-two times.

See how it goes, that's all you said to yourself. It's no big deal. Even if it doesn't work, just stay with her until you have sex. Time's pressing on – you're sixteen. You've checked her out since secondary school.

That's a terrible thought.

Stay with her until after Christmas then, so she's not upset over Christmas…

6

A hundred people gather round an arm-wrestling competition near the steps in the Maggy May. Some hang over the upper floor railings for a better view. The shouting builds and turns into a cheer when someone wins. Another competitor squeezes into the crowd, getting fired-up by his mates.

'You need to get in on that,' Ryan says to me, setting down the sweaty food he's brought over from the dinner hatch. 'Mr. Big Guns. Show them how it's done.'

Emma detaches herself from me and goes to a Psychology class. I've been secretly touching her butt under her brown skirt all morning.

'You two kiss *way* too much. People talk about it,' Ryan says.

'Okay.' I'm drawing in a sketch book with biro. 'It's just a phase.'

'It's not. She's obsessed over you. She's probably in fucking love with you. Seriously. You could cheat on her and she'd be like, "He didn't *mean* it." If you broke up with her, she wouldn't even come into college for a fortnight, I bet. It would ruin her.'

I huff, but that echo –

　　　… ruin her

　　　　　　　… ruin her

　　　… ruin her

　　　　　　　　　　– is hard to ignore. I'm strapped in.

My hand snakes into the right-hand zipped pocket of my back-pack for the tablets. I take some more paracetamol and a Stemetil and I don't think Ryan's noticed.

7

Me and Emma fool around upstairs at Ant's house party on his mum's bed. When we emerge downstairs a massive '*Waheeey!*' builds from the crowd. Ant later tells me the living room light had been swinging. Then Morgan potters through with his trousers down, a big meat knife pressed on the base of his cock. 'Tell me it's small or I'll cut if off,' he says.

'It looks alright to me,' I say.

'Tell me it's small or it's—'

'Jesus, fine, it's small.'

Emma saves a seat for me on the bus every morning, often wearing nice clothes that her friends will later murmur were to impress me. I have to pretend to be okay, make conversation and be funny, be close, kiss and touch on the ride home until one night the loud kids at the back shout, 'Give it a fucking rest.'

Emma pulls her cuff up to her palm and smears it over the window. I see the white and red spotlights on the British Oxygen tower shining on the exposed pipework spaghetti below, the lights of the steel distributors and mountains of scrap metal. Emma's coat smells like maggots. The tubs of them Dad would buy for bait when we used to go fishing. I don't know where the smell comes from: Emma herself smells nice. She hugs me as the bus grumbles into Barton; I catch that maggot scent under her collar and mouth 'What *is* that?!' to no one.

A month goes by and I've left college by lunch a dozen times now. Staying here a full day is hard enough, let alone dreading the ride home with Emma suffocating me. Why doesn't she sit with someone else for a change?

I'll say, 'Back in a sec,' and duck out the Maggy May, then keep walking all the way into town and onto a bus. Send Emma excuses via text why I disappear, even a lie or two. I don't keep track.

Guess where I am?xx, I write, as though loveably random, when really I've walked two miles to Tesco, just to get away from her.

One afternoon I'm sat upstairs on an early bus home, waiting for it to leave the station. I get a text from Emma announcing that she's coming too: could I ask the driver to wait two minutes? *Argh, damn. Sorry, we've already gone! xx*, I lie, looking about and hoping the bus will indeed set off.

I like her very much.

I get introduced to her family in a situation I make sure will have to be brief.

'Nice to meet you all,' I say in their council terrace lounge. The white innards of teddies, specks of rubber chews and the fibres of coloured rope their big dog has ripped to bits are trodden into the high carpet pile. Old wooden cabinets displaying glass bowls line the walls and close the room in. The sofas are covered in layers of throws and have white meal tables tucked up to their arms with laptops resting on them. The ceiling is thick with plaster patterns and the chandelier hangs low. Massive speakers, like you'd see in a teenage boy's room, are stacked against the free wall, between the TV and the two cages. In one cage is a hamster, in the other is a rat.

I sit very still on the arm of a sofa. Emma holds my hand with both of hers and puts her head on my thigh as though I'm staying.

'*He's* fit,' Emma's older sister mumbles to her mum. I pretend not to hear.

'I wish I could stop but my family are outside. We're off to my auntie's house.'

And off I go. In and out like an assassin.

8

The shimmer of TV colours through my eyelids pull me out of another dream where my family were returning to Florida.

I reach down and pat the carpet until I find the DVD remote. *Scrubs* season three is on, which I've seen in ten-minute pre-sleep snippets a dozen times through. Tonight, it's the episode where Turk eats a steak too fast. 'I'm sick to the stomach,' he suddenly declares in a restaurant, and I imagine the horror I'd feel in that situation. Stranger still is the scene where his girlfriend Carla takes care of him later on at home, rubbing his stomach and assuring him it's only indigestion. How can he let her stay with him, *touch* him, when he feels ill?

I turn the DVD player and TV off and wait to fall back to sleep.

I'm definitely at home. Here in my room, in bed, in Barton.

Nothing's forcing me to leave.

9

I take a full day off college, which leads into a second.

At twenty to eight I leave home, but instead of waiting at the bus stop, I keep going. Check no one I know can see me before hopping the picket fence into Top Field and walking on.

At the base of Death Hill, in the concrete ditch a quarter-full of frozen mud, I use sixty pence of precious phone credit to call in sick. A woman on the line asks what's wrong with me, which seems a bit rude. And then says she'll need a letter from my parents confirming it, which dashes all hope of getting away with this so I hang up.

Emma, my parents, teachers, the woman on the phone – everyone wants to know where I am.

In the field Death Hill overlooks, which once grew cauliflowers, where me and Ben smoked a pouch of Samson in the dark a few years ago, diggers now gouge foundation trenches for a housing development and pile up the soil in a mound. I find a patch of the ditch where thorny creepers haven't grown up and died. Sit down and rest my feet on an empty tin of baby formula. Watch the men in high-vis jackets go about their digging.

'What's this one?'

I swirl the blotchy red liquid about the shot glass and a drop slops over the lip.

'Chilli vodka,' comes the answer. 'It's fucking minging.'

It tastes vile after the mint and berry shots from a minute ago. I smack the empty glass down and wait for that quick shudder. Through the blurs of arms arranging drinks, smiles moving, I spot Emma across the room and watch her for a moment. I'm embarrassed that we couldn't arrive together, like couples should. She asked but I insisted on meeting her here. Like mates. I don't get why her request was so daunting.

Propped up in an old armchair, Boris is paralytic.

I get my digital camera out. 'Let me take a picture as though you're sober as a nun and, like, enjoying polite conversation,' I say.

Boris laughs, looks down at his limbs. Arranges one leg over the other. Lays one arm on the chair's arm, holds up his drink with the other. Puts on a concerned frown and nods slowly.

'Okay, now let me take a picture of how you actually feel.'

And he just goes 'Braaaagh!' and sprawls out, throws his drink up the wall and lollops his head back. 'I don't even know who I am,' he says to the ceiling, and falls asleep.

A dozen of us play Ring of Fire, and one poor girl has to drink a two-pint shit mix: everyone's drink poured into a deep glass measuring jug with added salt, brown sauce and tabasco. 'Fucking do it,' Ryan demands, after her nose hovers above it for too long. Then the bated silence as she chugs, and the '*awww*' as we see the glob of brown sauce that's settled at the bottom slip into her mouth.

There's a sound of retching but it isn't her. I turn to see Boris, still asleep with his head back, being sick down himself in that armchair like an erupting volcano.

My drawings in the Maggy May become a form of light entertainment friends check in on between lessons. I love using biro: the tiny precision strokes, the slow deepening of blacks as the layers are added. My head gets right down near the paper, back arched, fringe tickling my hand. I can fall into the detail, concentrating enough to quiet my need to flee college. Just a little bit. Just for a moment or two. 'It can take the edge off.'

Drawing gives me space to think about distances: between here and the bus stop, from the bus stop to home. I think about travel time: between now and the bus, now and home, between the areas of invisibility. Because there may be nowhere on the bus to hide, but beside the back roads are places I could disappear: hedgerows, naked now the leaves have fallen, but enough to obscure my identity to passers-by; ridges and ditches; garden walls and evergreen trees. But between these things are the wretched open fields and the busy streets in Scunthorpe.

Just try to concentrate on the shading of this tree.

Don't vomit right here on a high table.

Lessons are getting harder to show up to. I'm forever on the verge of hurling. Recurring daydreams haunt me – shape-shifting and undefined, like that old 'Walking in the Air' video done with squiggly crayon – of sprinting away from wherever I'm sat, coughing hot sick across clean clothes and carpet. I set timers on my phone that count down to five minutes after the lesson ends. No idea why this helps.

Scrutinise the layout of every classroom: distance between me and the door, number of people to manoeuvre past should I have to leave, how many face me where I'm sat and how many would face me if I made my way out. Number of people, full stop. Classroom density, you know? Is the teacher the understanding sort, or would he or she make a scene if I tried to go? All situations have an extremely strong *vibe*. Dense classrooms feel like cauliflower hearts and sparse, easy-to-leave classrooms feel like pushing empty bottles through the bristled hole of a recycle bin. Sometimes it feels like music or a film. To try and distract myself from the reel of images getting louder behind my eyes, I draw patterns down the margins of my notebooks: kites and grids, tentacles and branches, spikes, blocks and blobs, all entwined. I decide a point of light and start shading. After three warnings, one teacher threatens to make me leave if I continue, which in college is pretty embarrassing. 'I *am* listening, though,' I whisper. My stomach doesn't jettison buttered toast and Polos, but if I speak another word it will.

Class ends and I walk all the way out of Scunthorpe, down a farmer's track, over a little motorway bridge and towards the M18.

Clumps of muck stick to my shoes and even though it's December I sweat.

Now what?

10

'Are you coming with us tonight?' Emma's sister Miranda says. It's Saturday morning and me and Emma are accompanying her on the short walk from their house to Barrow's car garage.

'Don't know yet.'

'How can you not know? You're either coming or not.' She laughs. A sort of angry laugh.

'It's up to Chris,' Emma pants, those shorter legs struggling to keep pace. But she's been asking, too.

Emma's family wants to take me to Cleethorpes cinema with them, later. It will be a cramped drive, a long process of parking, queuing for movie tickets, her family and the cinema audience watching me run past them all to find a bathroom. I estimate times and distances, and wonder whether I could jump out the car, or call my parents for rescue from Cleethorpes. I've never been there, but there's a firm idea in my mind of how it'll play out, and what the cinema, the streets, the car park look like.

This makes for an awkward day. At Emma's house, I'm saying, 'Not sure,' to her dad one moment, hearing Miranda tell their brother, '*Chris* doesn't know if he's coming,' the next. Emma's clearly bursting to ask me again.

What gave them the fucking idea to invite me along?

In the evening, Emma's mother pokes her head into the bedroom where I kiss her daughter and asks me sweetly whether I'm coming.

'Not today,' I say, scrunching up inside.

Even more sweetly, 'Any particular reason?'

'Just don't really fancy it,' is the best I can manage.

The journey to Cleethorpes from Emma's house passes through Barton, so they offer to drop me off on their way. No one mentions my refusal to join them. Squished in the back seat, Emma's hand finds mine and strokes it. And as we leave the marketplace, past the fire station where one of the big square doors are open and the vacant interior is lit up a sterile white, and turn left to climb the road to my house, I'm on the brink of saying, 'Actually, just keep going. I'll come with you.' But the bravery is fleeting.

'Thanks for the lift,' I chirp as we pull up at my house. 'Have a great time.'

I sidestep between my parents' cars and pull my key out.

'"Have a great time"?' I repeat under my breath, unlocking the front door and watching their car turn round at the top of my road. I should be with them.

Emma is a ball and chain, but not like men say with a friendly elbow to each other's ribs. She's a responsibility that dangles off everything I have to do. Adding new things I have to do. **Seeing** everything I do. Clinging onto me like a koala bear that talks and wants to kiss and turn me on. Adding time limits. Removing spontaneity, which is all that lets me do anything. Even hanging out with friends is getting harder. And if letting Emma come round for an evening is enough to make me want to puke, how about jobs, kids, marriage? A massive, sprawling system of images I don't want to be a part of explodes. Journeys to work, meetings, romantic holidays, taking my children on a day out or being left with them, travelling long distances. Every situation pops into sub-images of me being ill, splits from trunks into branches into twigs. I daydream for hours, picturing it all and wondering if I'll be sick, here, there, today, tomorrow.

11

Perdita, Emma's dog, has died; I find out via text on the way home from college one night. Has it been ill for a while? My fingers drum the back of my Motorola Razor whilst I cook up a reply.

I open my front door an hour later and Emma runs in. I wave to her mum, who's pulling away. No one else is home: my parents are at work and Jordan's got a rugby presentation. I see Emma without make-up on for the first time and she looks really nice. She's red and swollen around the eyes. The sleeves of her jumper are pulled all the way over her hands. She dabs a teardrop that's come to the tip of her nose and I glimpse the bunched fingers inside her sleeve like a little hermit crab. Normally she takes off her scarf by now and hangs it on our banister but she forgets, so I help. I hold her for ages whilst she cries. It's quiet. She keeps her face in my chest for a while and then turns away so she can breathe.

12

Winter starts settling in. Emma comes over and we go straight upstairs to my room. Cuddle, make out and explore each other. It's our routine. Mum's had words with me about it.

'I'm *freezing*,' Emma says, starting to jump into my bed.

'No you don't,' I say. 'If you get in my bed, you're not allowed any clothes on. They're the rules.'

'Your rules?' She puts her hands on her hips, smiling. Strips down to her underwear. 'Now can I get in?'

I de-clothe and get in, too.

By the time we're touching each other, the sickness subsides. I get so turned on my body trembles.

'I'm just cold,' I explain, embarrassed and unsure whether that's true or not.

We later talk about how much we like each other, how we're ready to have sex.

One Sunday morning I'm halfway under my desk, re-arranging some wires so I can move my speakers.

The bedroom door opens enough for Dad's head to peer through.

'This new girlfriend of yours,' he says.

'Yeah?'

'Just be careful.'

'Oh. I will be. You don't have to tell me,' I say.

He nods and his head retracts. The door pulls to.

Me and Emma play *Gears of War* together on my Xbox and laugh at how frightened she gets when a monster storms in; she yells and her character spins in a hopeless circle before getting cut in half with the monster's chainsaw.

I walk into Barton's marketplace to get a haircut, which makes me nervous. It never used to. But it occurs to me that I'm obliged to stay for the whole job, even if I suddenly become sick, unless I run out with half-cut hair and look like a tool. Sat waiting for my appointment to start, I estimate how long the haircut should take. Twenty minutes? Could I hold myself together for that long if a sickness came over me? Emma sends a text from my bedroom saying the game's scaring her. It's scaring me that she's there playing it. When I get home, I find her cross-legged on the bed, reading her book. She eyes up my hair.

'Well?' I say. 'I mean, he's not styled it the way I would, so it'll look better after a shower.'

'It looks…' she scrunches her mouth and nods, 'different.'

'Different! Thanks a lot. Different.'

'I'm not saying *bad*,' she laughs, but I tackle her onto her back before she can say any more.

We make out for what must be an hour; I run downstairs to get us a drink, past Jordan panic-clicking off the porn he's watching on the family computer, which I pretend not to notice.

'Have you ever been in love?' Emma asks. We're back in bed; she faces away and I've got my arm around her.

'Yeah.'

'Sophia?'

'Yeah,' I say.

'Did nothing ever develop there?'

'No, it all went to pot.'

'Do you still love her?'

'No, of course not.' I squeeze Emma.

My hand reaches beneath her underwear the first time whilst *Scrubs* plays on my bedroom TV. She makes little gasps and sighs into my mouth as my fingers enjoy her until my forearm burns. Emma uses her hand on me and before I can stop her I come all over my t-shirt.

'I don't know what to do,' I say, looking down at myself when the haze has cleared.

'Put it in the wash? I wouldn't wear it to dinner, anyway.'

'I can't put it in the wash. It's weird.'

There's an old cutlery suitcase on top of my cupboard that only I know the code to. I pull it down and stuff the sticky t-shirt into it, on top of the old *Jackass* tapes me and my friends made when we were twelve, the CD-ROMs of downloaded porn Morgan used to deal out, and the crispy pair of boxers I had a wet dream in a couple of years back. I clip the locks shut and put it back on the cupboard. Emma laughs. I kiss her.

'You coming for tea?' James shouts from downstairs. 'We're having *soup*!'

'Well, do you want *soup*?' I say quietly, and Emma's laughing even more.

We go downstairs, the light stinging our eyes in the hall, and through to the kitchen. 'We're having *soup*!' Emma says to James.

'Is that how I said it?' He smiles, sawing a stick bread.

Emma wants to fit in with my family. Even Jordan, who can barely say a word when she's around.

Dad arrives as Mum's putting soup in the bowls. It's eight o'clock; he's at the end of another sixteen-hour day. Dad manages a company owned by his brother-in-law Lowell Hobart, that makes and fits windows. For weeks now they've been working at Lincoln prison and he has to be there at the crack of dawn. 'Hi, love,' he says when he spots Emma.

Me and Emma tuck into our dinner, rosy-cheeked and nudging each other. The next day at college we're all the closer, whispering about the night before into each other's ear. Then I escape home early.

Everyone is obliged to attend two extracurricular lessons a week and I haven't been to one yet. And I can rarely bring myself to go to the double Media lesson on Thursday afternoons anymore. I find an email about my attendance slipping.

At night whilst I'm delivering newspapers, a text arrives from Emma, letting me know she can't stop thinking about me. *There's something I really want to tell you*, she writes. Like I don't know.

13

I make it to the computer room for Tutorial. My personal tutor sits beside me, and his army-green jumper looks too warm. He lays out some paper with register tables on it and quietly asks, 'How are we getting on then, Chris?' There are gaps everywhere in the little boxes that mark my attendance.

'You know,' I trail off. 'I've not been well recently.'

14

It's Tuesday in the last half-week before the Christmas holidays. I only meant to take Monday off this week: I couldn't face the bus, face Emma, everyone else that could see me, the journey, the long day of loud crowds and quiet classrooms.

A pattern's developing where I wuss out and skip the bus, feel relieved but ashamed, promise I'll go in tomorrow for *sure*. Then tomorrow comes around and a reason not to go will emerge. But *tomorrow's* different. I *must* go in. After all, I took last Wednesday through Friday off.

But now James gets a stomach bug.

I tread around the house trying not to touch anything, breathing shallow when I'm near a room James is in or has been in. Shut my bedroom door and lean out the window so the cold air touches my tongue. At dinner I wish I knew which knives and forks he's used in the last month. But they're all fucking identical.

'It just came over me out of nowhere!' James says as cheerfully as remembering a laughing fit. 'Pretty sure I'm alright, now.'

'Should I wake him up?' I hear Mum ask Dad later, whilst James sleeps on the sofa. 'He wouldn't want to be there, if, you know…'

You know? Know what?

'He's fine,' Dad says.

I lie awake in the night wondering when the illness will strike me. On the journey to Leggott, in front of Emma? In a class, in the dead silence? In the Maggy May, in front of thousands? News will spread like wildfire. I'll get a name. At what point would I have been contaminated, and how long until the symptoms begin? Oh God I can't work it all out. Was it the cup I used that James used the day before he came down with it, in what they call the "incubation period"? Or the moment earlier today, when I opened his bedroom door to ask if he needed some water?

Better to just not go into college.

This term is a write-off.

I fall asleep worrying how I'll pass the year.

With freezing thumbs I write a text to Emma from the end of a tractor route that splits two fields on the outskirts of Barton. *Can't believe I haven't seen you for a week now! Miss you loads xxx*

I look around for signs of life.

No one.

My parents are both at work by half eight, so normally it's safe to head home shortly after. But with James there, I should wait a little longer. At least until it seems like I've been on a half day.

The trenches from tractor tyres are furred with frost, but as the sunshine moves over the southern field's bump it starts to disappear and the mud gives under my feet. I pace about, find somewhere to lean, pace some more.

The grandfather clock would *chick-chock* at my grandparents' when I'd have a day off primary school sick. Lying on their sofa, the only thing to do was listen to it. Hear it *bong* the hours in, hear it get wound.

Ten o'clock passes and the cold starts getting to me. I walk home. The last road before our street is always dicey: it's the main way in from the dual carriageway, from Hull, Scunthorpe, Grimsby, the sort of places my parents patrol. If they see me without me knowing and then later hear my story about being at college, it would expose this secret. I walk quick and scrutinise every car for a familiar face.

Very carefully, I creep under our windows, working my way round the back and into the muddy side alley where no one goes. Lean against the wall and listen to the pipe which I know comes out from the living room. Tuck my jumper into my trousers, my scarf inside my jumper, pull my coat as tight as it goes, but the shivering won't stop. I dig a bucket out the pile of rubble back here, turn it upside down on the mud and sit, hugging my torso. A long hour passes; perhaps it's time for some lunch. The orange I've packed myself is difficult to peel with stiff fingers. And my hands, which aren't sufficiently washed, must not touch the fruit's flesh. I loosen enough rind with my mouth to pinch between two fingers. Pull more with my teeth. I manage to guide a sour segment out with my lips and tongue but then drop the whole lot. Bright orange on hard, black mud. Kick it away. One slice is enough. Too much fruit might upset the stomach, anyway. I wonder whether the fumes of James's illness can seep out of that pipe in the wall. Open my bag again and pull out *Cat on a Hot Tin Roof*, which we're studying in Literature class. Better to be productive at least. I read a few pages but the cold doesn't let me concentrate.

'What're you doing home?' James says, making himself breakfast.

I've given up and gone inside.

'Only had one lesson with it being the last day.'

'Really?'

'No.' I sigh and drop onto a kitchen chair. Already my hands throb.

'Have you been to *any* lessons?'

'No.'

I get ready for him to ask, *Then… where have you been?*

'That's alright,' is all he says.

'It's not. I'm barely going at all. Mum and Dad don't know.'

'Want a tea?' He suspends a second bag over a mug. Drops it in when I nod.

Over Christmas I manage to go to Emma's once or twice. Throw some presents at her and get the hell out.

15

G irl one: 'Are you off tonight?'
Girl two: 'What's it called again?'
Girl one: 'Barton on Humber.'

My ears prick up in Literature class, but I pretend I'm still writing about pantheism and letters from Africa. It's spring, 2007.

They're obviously on about the same party I'm going to. Hearing Barton mentioned by anyone outside our circle of friends is like seeing someone you know on TV. I have it on good authority those two talking are from Doncaster, forty-five miles from the party. The host, Cassandra, a girl I know from school, is trying to get elected for Student Council, whatever that entails, and is gunning for votes via popularity. Popular is one thing she's not. I knew our group was going tonight, but apparently word's spreading through the college. I bite into my Polo.

'A couple of strangers were talking about Cassy's,' I tell Ben in the Maggy May after class.

'Same.' He leans over his box of chicken. 'I heard people mention it in Biology just now. If it spreads too far, there'll be *loads* of people there tonight. It's turning into something you'd see on *The fucking O.C.*' By which he means an American TV drama he hates, including unrealistically massive house parties with red cups held aloft, girls jumping into blue-lit pools, nerds getting turned away at the door, beer kegs brought in on the shoulders of football players. All that bollocks. Our house parties are more like six or seven of us getting quietly drunk looking into a fire pit, smoking a pack of fags and ordering a Pizza Jim's, and we wouldn't trade it.

I meet up with Emma and we walk into town. She buys a sausage roll and I flip through the music in HMV until the bus arrives and we take the hour's trip to my house.

No one's at home and we're soon kissing and undressing each other in my bedroom.

'I wish we could have sex, so much,' Emma says whilst my fingers make a beckoning gesture under her thong.

A thought strikes me and I stop. 'We *could*! We've got a couple of Johnnies. Ant gave me a dodgy one he got in Turkey but the other's a Durex.'

She looks very happy. 'Okay.'

And so, like the instructional lesson at school taught me, I roll a condom down myself and we have sex for the first time. Quarter of an hour or so in, whilst Emma is having a try on top of me, Mum rings.

'Eugh, you're *answering*?' Emma laughs.

I press the green button. Unaware what Mum's talking about, I just say, 'Ah right, yep, yep, okay.'

Emma moves her hips. I poke her tummy, mouthing, 'Stop it'.

I hang up.

'Sorry about that,' I say. Though I'm not *that* sorry: a momentary turn-off will surely make me last longer.

A few minutes later, I say something to encourage Emma. She's moving on top of me, hands holding mine. 'It feels so good.'

'Really?' she says. Her expression shows relief, like she was worried I hadn't been enjoying it at all. A sort of crooked smile, looking down at me with a bit of perspiration on her forehead. It's a moment I know I'll never forget, although it's hard to know why. It's her face. That 'Really?' floating in a fast exhale. Not knowing that her face is a bit skewed with either exertion or pleasure. I fall in something like love. Is it love? Or do I just feel immensely sorry for her? The heartfelt investment in that face, that 'Really?', and the earnest search into my eyes for reciprocation. Maybe it's her love I feel, even though we've already exchanged our promises of love a few weeks ago whilst kissing to Radiohead's 'How to Disappear Completely', of all songs. Maybe I've fallen in sympathy. My investment is in the love she's giving, not in her. Or maybe I do love her. Now isn't the time to wonder.

Evening arrives and we head to the party. It makes me uncomfortable to go together but it feels inappropriate not to, given what we've just done. I'm a new level of involved now. Our sex was a sweaty contract signing.

In the 1998 version of *The Man in the Iron Mask* is a moment that disturbed the fuck out of me as a child. Louis XIV, King of France, listens to his twin brother beg for death rather than be forced to put back on the hideous, heavy iron mask. Louis then orders him to wear it for the rest of his life, and above his brother's anguished moans as the mask is locked back on his head, screams, "Wear it until you *love* it!"

Jesus, poor Emma. What a thing to liken her to. No, it's just the "until you love it" line that's reared its head. If I don't love her now, I will eventually.

We're heading up Caistor Road, renowned for its crime. It's dark now, with just a hint of orange left in the sky, and a warm breath of wind for March. I've got Emma's hand in mine. I stop us for a moment and we make out. She then holds my hips and does a happy little wiggle, beaming up at me.

'Can you hear that?' I ask. 'Surely that's not the party.'

Emma bends a corner of her mouth down. 'I reckon it is.'

Cassandra's place must be half a mile away and already distant screams, cheers and the deep thud of a kick drum float in the air above the sound of traffic, like we're on our way to a street carnival or rock concert.

'News just in. Disaster's struck. The trampoline is broken. Bare metal – snappage,' Ant reports to my camera, holding his beer as a pretend microphone. 'Oh, and news just in… *Party's fucking banging!*'

The four-metre-across trampoline gets hoicked up on its side like a giant coin and rolled across the back garden. Over the perfect lawn, down a step and over the bamboo flower garden, hitting the shed. Everyone scatters out the way as it goes. It finally tips, landing on the conservatory, and with the sound of cracking plastic the gutter comes down. A metal leg and a hand of springs dangle off the trampoline.

Cassandra has a big house but there are *hundreds* here, more than she possibly could've expected. A few dozen aren't even from college, I know that for a fact. People are out on the lawn scrunching up used cans and throwing them over the fence or at an upstairs window; they're down in the lower patio, sat on the backs of the deckchairs smoking, and someone's squeezing into the coal bunker; they're up on the deck beneath the creepers and solar-powered lamps; in the conservatory having a go on her dad's gym equipment; they're crammed down the corridors and the cream carpets are muddied; they're playing drinking games in the kitchen and dining room; the rugby teams have commandeered the lounge and they're into notoriously weird shit so I stay out; people are slipping upstairs; cheap cars are revving out front; someone takes a run-up and shoulders straight through the octagonal summerhouse wall, then its whole roof collapses to a massive cheer. I haven't seen Cassandra yet. Her parents went out for a meal and a drink, letting their daughter have the house for a little get-together, and are apparently due home by one. The place is getting wrecked.

'Who cares. She's *rich*,' I overhear one girl say.

I put my camera in Emma's handbag; there are too many strangers to take pictures without looking like a weirdo.

Ben checks the soles of his shoes.

'I feel like I've trod in shit,' he says, sniffing the air.

In a moment where it's just me, him and Ryan, I say, 'Guess what? I've sealed the deal.'

'Shit!' Ben plucks my top. 'Chris went home a boy and returns a man.'

'I lasted thirty-five minutes,' I say.

Ryan, now the last remaining virgin of the Three Musketeers, doesn't say much. He hops the fence into Dog Park to take a piss and a minute later Ben chases him, chanting, 'Ryan's got his cock out,' and forcing Ryan to run away mid-stream.

The sock salesman George is still shagging arrives in a suit that's way too big. His ink-blue trousers bunch up on his polished shoes; he's opened the first couple of buttons of his shirt and from the fold beneath his double chin emerges a thin gold necklace holding a small amulet. It doesn't go down well. You hear the odd murmur of 'Has the girl's dad come home?' or just 'Who's the wanker in a suit?' but he's oblivious and talks about target audiences and unique sales propositions with anyone who'll listen.

Maybe they finally get a word in and ask, 'So what's your product?'

'Socks.'

We find a second lounge with a massive library of records and an antique piano in the corner. Ben lifts its lid with his wiry arms. Places his alcopop on the music rack. Stares down at the keys and swipes his fingers up and down them, making that noise from old TV shows, where the screen goes wobbly before a dream sequence begins. It must hurt his fingers. Then he starts to play 'Black and White Rag'. Heads turn and I see their lips say, 'Is that real?' 'Oh my god.' A bunch of others arrive to see who's doing it. 'Fucking hell, I thought that was a CD playing.'

A guy lines up a footstool, shouts, '*Fucking...*', jumps off and grabs the light to swing from it, but his weight rips the shade straight off and the bulb blows up, leaving us in near-darkness. He lands on his heels, which slip on the carpet, and he slams onto his back.

'I've got door handles,' a voice says in my ear.

It's Wykes, stood in the light coming in from the hall. He lifts his hoody up and opens his pocket; it's full of cutlery.

'You said door handles,' I say.

'I've stashed them outside.'

'How'd you get them off?'

'Twenty pence,' he says, pulling the coin out and demonstrating a screwing action. It's then I notice that even the door to the room we're in has a hole where the handles used to be.

'But why? *Why?*' The more I think about it, the more I laugh.

A different tone starts percolating through the house. Scrunched noses and the odd person shrieking and running outside.

I'm back in the crowded kitchen, and it's a bomb site. Empty bottles and cans line every surface. Dregs dribble off the counters, into the drawer cracks, down the cupboards. Muddy footprints, leaves, more bottles, even broken coal briquettes are scattered across the tiled floor. Ben comes to find me.

'It's not my shoe.'

'Eh?'

'One of the rugby cunts,' he says, between disgust and admiration. 'They've taken a shit and hidden it somewhere in the house.'

People are catching wind and more are emptying into the already crammed garden.

'Have you seen Cassy?' I ask.

Ben shrugs.

She's not seen at college for nearly a week.

16

Apparently. Because I'm not there either.

I walk along the chalk path overlooking Pebbly Beach, down by the Humber. It's sunny. Maybe that's what tipped the scales and stopped me going to college today. Sunshine means exposure, high visibility, heat. Heat leads to headaches, and headaches lead to vomiting and diarrhoea. Not that I'm a doctor. When summer arrives it will be even hotter and the days even longer.

And there are three AS exams to sit at the end of term. Each one is three hours long. The thought drags a clangour of images along with it like tin cans bouncing behind a newlyweds' limo. I'm almost stopped in my tracks. It must be the hundredth time I've thought about the exams since getting up two hours ago, but there's no getting used to it.

Three hours, three times.

Lately, everything I do gets measured next to three hours. I make a note of a time and set an alarm on my phone for three hours later. When the alarm rings, I ask myself how long it felt. I might compare a part of my day to the length of a *Lord of the Rings* film. If I need the bathroom, I'll see if I can hold it in for three hours. How can an illness deepen in three hours? At any given time in the day I will stop, check the time, and wonder what I was doing three hours ago, and how long ago that feels. What journeys take three hours that I might compare the exams to? I could take the bus to college, the bus home, and the bus to college again. I could walk to Hull in that time, I think, glancing over the Humber now, to that little white hotel my cousin got married in. I've got to come to terms with **three hours**.

Exams are a massive problem. Always have been.[2] The silence, the volume of people, being unable to leave. I was bricking it all the way up to last year's GCSE exams. Not because I cared if I did well, but because they were mandatory. You *had* to sit in that hall, in sight of your year group, for hours at a time. No one could escape the exams. Our head of year would threaten to come knock on doors if you didn't show up. Waiting outside the sports hall before the first exam, watching a group of lads play football with a dead blackbird, it struck me how easy it would be to start stepping backwards, turn and walk away, leave my future behind. I didn't do well in half the exams because I was too concerned whether I could make it through. And in the depths of quiet, one girl – renowned for weirdness but also intelligence – got up and ran out the sports hall, beginning to sob. The footsteps were loud and reverberated. I heard clothes rubbing and chair plastic bending: a mass stillness stirred as a couple of hundred people turned at their little tables to watch her. From behind the breezeblock wall where the changing rooms were came the sound of retching.

And look at me now.

If I can't make it to a standard day at Leggott, a few lessons, how will I possibly make it to these coming exams? The thought of going

---

[2] Little memories of primary school SATs tests. How long did I dread them? How frightened did I feel in Bowmandale hall, a little bean of a boy hunched over his maths questions? The metallic dust smell of piano strings nearby, the nauseating gravy and custard smell that still hung in the air from dinner.

to college today floods me even now, even though I've not gone. Vivid daydreams: what might have been, what might yet be. Just like last night and this morning. Just like yesterday morning. Yes, a broken record. I picture myself needing to be sick. The faces who see me on the bus. In the classroom. The expressions. The fucking whispers. Text messages spreading like a virus. Judgement. That wait in the Maggy May between lessons. Drawing to keep the vomit down. But I'm not in control of my body. It carries me around and I'm at its mercy. It chooses if it wants to shame me. Emma. Taste of butter and the sight of soggy bread. Me not wanting to eat. The long wait on the bus when it stops in town. Its complete halt at every bus stop and the agonisingly slow acceleration once it sets off again, whilst I silently beg it to hurry the fuck up. Oh God when the doors close. The places I can hide by the road. The time between them. Kisses. Me jetting fluids from mouth and ass. Like shooting a bouncy castle that's full of minestrone soup. The smell of the bus. The tablets in my bag. My pocket. More painkillers. Does this hurt my liver? Will that make me sick? Will it happen in public? 'It just came over me out of nowhere!' Whole fat milk glugging from the bottle. Feeling it go down. Mixing with tuna flakes and citrus fruit in my stomach. Children being sick and shitting themselves cross-legged on the carpet in primary school and we form a circle around them. Breathing in other people's breath. A drumroll. Emma telling me 'It's okay.' Me being smelled. A cubicle door. Raising my hand to be excused from class. The time it takes to leave. Do I grab my books, or leave everything? Is my stomach audible? My clothes. The perfumes and hair products of the girls. My deodorant slowly lost in the stench of my own filth. Pot Noodle splashed over the pavement. Spreading words.

'Morning,' I say to another walker. Her Jack Russell touches my trousers with its nose as it skips past on the chalk.

There's a low concrete wall between the path and the rocky slope down to the silt and brown water. I walk along it for a while, careful of the bramble vines that have grown over it and died. When my feet disturb a tuft of long grass stalks, a couple of insects that were cozied up in there fly away and a dandelion head floats out, breaking into its little black-tipped parachutes.

The more immediate problem today is the university convention at college tonight. There's a talk from our headmaster at quarter past seven for twenty minutes and then we can mooch about the stalls and talk to representatives from different universities. Our invitation came in a brown envelope addressed directly to my parents, disguised amongst the bills and adverts. Just another brown envelope. Maybe I would've intercepted the letter and burned it if I'd known. I've read and re-read its simple schedule. Twenty-minute talk. Parents having questions at the end, no doubt. Metal chairs arranged closely together to make escape difficult without asking your row to stand up and let you past, I bet. Could we secure an aisle seat? The chances aren't good. Images bark at me: feeling sick, needing to leave, shitting myself. I see my parents driving me there; they'll take the motorway, not the back roads like the bus takes. Motorways mean driving at high speed; it will take longer to halt if I need to get out the car, assuming my parents would stop. Ducking out, onto the hard shoulder, I'll be visible from six lanes. There's a comfort in that most of the journey is lined with high banks, thick with trees and bushes to hide in, and given the current sunset time of about eight o'clock, it might be a *little* dark on the way there, or the sun might be low enough to obscure the eyes of some people looking my way; but several sections of the motorway run through flat, empty land, where you can see the industrial end of Brigg, a mile in the distance, and I will be visible to anyone over there with half-decent eyesight when I hop the barrier. What would the chances be, if I ask Dad to pull the car over, that we happen to halt in a spot where I'm visible from Brigg? Would he understand if I then said, 'Actually, can you scoot the car up another two hundred yards?'

Our headmaster has that photographic memory. Apparently, before a new year group starts, he has a flick through a big file of names and ID photos, and that's it: every name learned. He knows mine. If I stood up to leave in the middle of his speech tonight, would he say, 'Where are you going, Chris?' The audience would learn my name right before I vomit everywhere.

The reeds are tall, splayed here and there by empty beer kegs, full bin bags and sofas. The silt has climbed all the way up the rocky beach, where as kids we'd look for globs of iron and ammonite fossils.

I turn back. Walk down the tree-tunnel stretch of Farrings Road, up Gravel Pit, where there's no path and cars tear right past me at full speed down the hill. I cut through the subway, catching the smell of rubber, then up my estate. I see the back windows of my house and hope Mum isn't there, looking out. Round the street corner, I peek down our row of houses: no cars on the drive. No one's here.

Being home when I'm not meant to be is like that feeling I got as a kid when I'd be awake past bedtime.

I plug James's bass guitar in and mess with the amp distortion, twang and bend the guitar's coiled wires, then let it trail off until there's only that faint buzz of the amp. It goes *plock* when I turn it off, and then the house is quiet. I can hear the living room clock, even from up here.

My parents arrive home after five. At the dinner table, they ask what I've been up to at college. And like most evenings, I have to lie.

No one mentions the uni convention. Is there a chance they've forgotten?

Dad pushes his chair back, leans over the table to gather up the plates.

'We'll get washed up and have a quick tea and then make a move,' Mum says to me.

Adrenaline tremors down my limbs. The reasons not to go close in fast again. Louder this time. Images, images, images. Again and again like a cartoon mallet to the head.

Nausea bobs up to the surface. How can it, so quickly?[3] Had it ever gone away?[4] Was it something we were just eating? That I ate earlier? I must be getting sick. It swirls and churns. What do

---

[3] 'He was *struck* with sickness,' I imagine someone saying about me. '*Struck* with sickness.'

[4] The Radiohead track '2+2=5' is suddenly at full volume in my head: "You have not been paying attention, paying attention, paying attention, paying attention. You have not been paying attention, paying attention, paying attention, paying attention." It's true, I haven't.

I do? Announce it at the table? Tell Mum privately and hope she understands?

My ears are burning in my hands. It's the evening. I'm sat here at my desk, elbows on my knees, holding my head. Listening to Mum and Dad. The bedroom door bursts open but I don't think Dad sees me jump. I'm sixteen, I mustn't show him I'm afraid.

'What's going on?' he says. And then, like a clap or a jab, '*Chris.*'
'I can't go.' Nor can I look up to face him.

The sighed profanity and the brush of the door over the carpet can't be told apart. The door slams and my coat falls off. Big footsteps going over the landing and into his room. Mum's voice. Something else banging. Big footsteps coming back. I brace. The door opens part way, a coat sleeve getting caught under it like brakes applying. He forces it the rest of the way; the top hinge complains and my coat stretches.

Silence for a second. '*Why?*' he jabs.
'I just... I don't know—'
'*What?*'
'I don't feel well.'
'Chris, get ready. *Move.*'
'I can't.'
Silence. Goes out and comes in.

'You "don't feel well". You're fine to go to the gym and drink that protein shit and go out with your mates and your girlfriend whenever it pleases you, but when it's something important, here we are.'

'It's not like that.'

'Then let's go!' And when I don't move, he says, 'You know what? I've had it. Do as you like. You're letting it slip away, aren't you?'

'I *want* to go. I just *can't.*'

He's gone.

'Wayne,' I hear Mum call from their bedroom.

'No,' he says, heading down the stairs. 'I've had it. I don't know why we waste our energy trying with him. He's not bothered.' He goes on and it's too muffled to hear now but I get the gist.

I'm furious that he thinks I pick and choose when to feel ill, and I want to chase him downstairs, stretch open one of his red ears and shout down it why he's wrong. But the more angry I get, the more my jaw locks shut. And the more I want to speak, the more my stomach wants to squeeze hot sick up my throat. My door's open, and over the landing, Mum's door is too. I know she's sitting as still as me.

Dried paint plasters the desk's surface – layers of different colours splotching out from perfect right angles of nothingness, where a canvas was laid down and worked on. I take a biro from my mug of pens and start shading a purple-grey stream of paint; the little desk wobbles under my arm. I check the time, check my stomach.

Am I ill yet?
No.
Am I ill yet?
No.

Highlight that with the mouse curser. Click copy. Hold down the paste key, watch it *scroooooooll* down over ten pages, fifty pages.

Any second, the answer might change. Any second now.

It's a twenty to thirty-minute drive to college. We've missed the head teacher's talk but the uni stands will be out a while longer. I've got to get there. I've *got* to. I pick myself up and go through to Mum's room. She's sat on the floor, against the radiator, in a little gap between the far side of the bed and the front window. She's no doubt upset, but that's not why she's sat down there; she sits there all the time.

'Come on, then,' I say quietly. 'But just us.'

'Why not Dad?' She then sighs. 'Fine.'

We go out of Barton, down the dual carriageway. I count ten minutes. We turn right at the Barnetby roundabout and onto the motorway. I look out my window the whole way. Maybe Mum talks to me, and maybe I answer, but I'm not aware of it. The sickness foams. Flotsam and froth licking the silt shore of a stagnant lake.

That little grip on my neck. The bumps in the road. I glance at the Fiesta's radio clock: it's been nearly twenty minutes and we're only just coming off the motorway to descend into Scunthorpe. I picture every roundabout, straight and traffic light-controlled junction we've yet to pass, and try to work out how much longer we'll be.

The illness moves.

A stir in my guts.

A stir.

Now a squeeze.

It is new and terrifying.

No, no, not the other end. This can't happen.

There's no toilet anywhere near here.

Panic buzzes under the skin. Images fly off the reel.

No toilet. Insides cramping. No toilet. Skin prickling.

Am I ill yet?

Yes you are.

Yes you are.

Yes you are.

I scan hedgerows and barriers more frantically than ever. All the cars going past us on the other side of the road, the ones we overtake and the ones that overtake us. All those watching eyes. I will have to jump out the car and shit by the kerb. We're going down the main ring road, barely at forty miles an hour. I look at the sun. Open the emergency compartment of my bag and start munching on Imodium tablets, some paracetamol and Stemetil, trying not to let Mum see what I'm doing. Watch a traffic light we're approaching. Please stay green. Oh, please.

It turns to red and we stop.

'We need to turn round.'

No answer.

'*Mum.*'

'We're not off back, Chris.'

'Mum, we need to go back *now*. I'm ill. Seriously. Mum? You've *got to turn round*.' It would be twenty minutes back, though. I get a better thought. 'Can you take us to Tesco?' Better to be ill there than college. 'Please?'

'For God's sake, you're not ill, Chris.' The lights turn green and off we go.

'I can't believe it. I'm asking you,' I say.

'Shut up. All the hell you've played up tonight. You're not sick and you can bloody lump it if you are.'

We keep going.

'I'll never forget this. That you won't listen to me when I'm this desperate. I won't forget this.' The only person in the world I trust and she's betraying me. I'm trapped and the car won't stop. I reach for the door handle. We're going at forty-five. Fuck it. I'll land alright.

But the squeezing in my stomach has eased. The tablets, have they saved me? They can't work that quick. Am I okay? A wash of warm ecstasy up my arms, down my legs. Maybe I'm okay. My armpits are wet but I'm cold. I let go of the handle. Mum hasn't noticed; she's pulling us into the reserve car park at college, furious with me still. I don't know why but I half expected her to go through this transformation with me and feel okay now, too.

As we head inside, the illness comes on again and I keep swallowing. We pass students with parents, students in their own cliques, holding prospectuses and looking happy. Talking, laughing. We go around the stalls. I don't know if I say anything, or if Mum's near me, or if she's saying anything. Prospectuses seem to be the medals of attendance so at some stalls I just take one and move on. I've got prospectuses on subjects I don't take from universities I haven't read the name of. The other students and parents talk enthusiastically about their life goals to the reps who wear bright polo tops and badges. I lean through, grab a handful of leaflets and go to another stall. The illness comes and goes. I'm barely aware of what we're doing. I know I ask Mum again if we can go to Tesco before going home, secretly wanting to be left there forever, until I'm better. But she has none of it. She's found some info too and is gripping it tight. Before I know it we're on the road home again, and I don't know how long we were there or who I spoke to. My bag's full of books, leaflets, free pens. Mum doesn't speak to me. I repeat my astonishment that she wouldn't turn round or take me to Tesco. The illness stops peaking.

17

Next morning, Emma sends a text: she isn't coming in until a later bus. This is enough encouragement to get me on the 07:50 outside my street. I'm surprised at myself.

It's the first time I've stepped on and not spotted Emma smiling at me, picking up the work binders she lays on the seat beside her to save it for me. I find an empty seat beside a stranger and relish being anonymous. There's just the girl I went out with in primary school who sits at the back, who I hope doesn't remember me. And that skinny, witch-like girl with the one-sided smile Emma sometimes talks to. And, of course, Sophia will be upstairs.

Thirteen minutes into the commute, depending on how many stops we make in Ferriby, the bus turns off the main road and rattles past a farm.

I spot a hare sprinting down one of the ploughed furrows, barely a different shade than the dust it kicks up.

The road is so rough that the patchwork of metal floor plates clank and slide over each other where the rivets have worked loose; a little trapped water escapes from one of the cracks, zigzags down the edges of a couple of plates, and drops into another gap.

Winteringham is a little village by the estuary. The first few gardens are on tall walls above us like we're entering via the bed of a canal. The bus pulls in at the corner opposite the newsagents and pub. Skull Lady gets on, pulling herself up the two stairs. Her hand, not so much shaking as veering all over like a fly, finds her coat pocket and produces a laminated pass. She holds it up to the driver – not that he can possibly read a word it says.

Skull Lady's face is fixed in a teeth-bearing grimace, her Basset Hound eyes sunken and sore, showing the flesh beneath her eyelids. She must be passing one hundred.

The driver nods at her card and she heaves her little trolley up from the pavement, shuffles a few feet down the aisle, slowly rounds the pole, hunched over and preparing herself to sit. Her vertebrae show, even through the coat. Her knees wobble in anticipation, then *plonk*, she drops into the seat. Holds the bar in front of her like her life depends on it. Her twiggy wrists stick out of her sleeves; all the bones in her hand are visible: pale tracks and bumps tied with black veins. Her head slowly turns this way and that, grimacing. Is she looking out the windows? Or at the adverts plastered above them, showing the statistical dependability of the contraceptive implant? Or the mounting number of young people, loud and foul-mouthed, now filling every seat, standing down the aisle and crouching on the stairs?

From my seat I see the driver's eyes in his interior mirror, watching until she's seated before driving us off. He turns left at the newsagents and we gather speed out the village, between rapeseed fields. I watch the Humber Bridge shrink behind the cement works. This section of the journey is the halfway point in terms of **distance**, but only a third of the way in terms of **time**.

In Scunthorpe's brick maze, I search out the window for shops open this early that might have a bathroom, alley ways with industrial-sized bins to hide between or even inside, the mini porches cut into the sheer walls, even the headstones in the graveyard. Would I be visible to passing cars? To pedestrians? To the top deck of this bus, where Sophia sits?

The bell dings as we pass between the cinema and car park to stop in the station. A pair of dole mums get off and wander into the shops. I wish I could join them, rather than sit still here another moment. The doors close; the driver reaches forward and yanks the steering wheel round.

'Hang on!' I shout, pulling an earphone out to hear the kids at the back shouting the same and dinging the bell. Skull Lady hasn't even finished turning herself to face the aisle. She puts a hand on the seat in front, a hand on her trolley, pulls herself once and fails. Pulls again.[5] Once she's as vertical as her body will go, she transfers

---

[5] I daydream of yelling, 'Jesus!' Scooping her tiny frame up and standing her down on the pavement outside. Saying, 'Let's bloody go,' to the driver, getting back in my seat and putting my earphone back in.

her second hand onto her trolley. Makes the treacherous journey to the door.

God. I wouldn't step a foot out the house if I was as slow as that. I know I can run fast and for a long time, climb things, slip into tight spaces, hide from the sights of others, if I need to. And that's a comfort for me. Often I watch disabled people getting pushed along in a wheelchair, propping themselves up with a walking stick, getting on the special bus or folding their scooter equipment into the boot of a custom-designed people carrier, knowing I couldn't show myself like they do. Unable to skip away. How does Skull Lady do it? I was concerned about the broad daylight coming through my curtains when I first opened my eyes this morning; I get nervous to carry my massive art folder about in case it slows me down or makes me too conspicuous in an emergency.

With a small measure of pride I make it to college, but I don't stay the whole day. Nor attend one lesson. In fact, once the bus drops us off, I wait until anyone who might know me has gone away and then head back to the station to go home. Before I become ill. Before Emma gets here.

I haven't been to Thursday's Media Studies since Christmas. I can't handle that two-hour free period wait beforehand, left in the Maggy May to think about the coming lesson, up all those stairs where it's stifling, and the bus ride home with Emma.[6] I started going home at dinner time instead, then I started going home straight after first period Literature. Now, it seems I don't go in on Thursdays at all. My momentary braveness this morning has come to nothing since I didn't sign in to one lesson. I might as well have stayed in Barton. Truth is, last night won't stop replaying. Dad forcing the door open with the *one, two*, the coat caught between it and the carpet. The '*Why?*' questions. How the sickness dropped from my stomach to my guts for no reason. Mum not turning round when I begged her.

The sugary smell of rotting garbage blows through an open window of the bus as it drags itself out of Scunthorpe. Daffodils by the road flare bright yellow in another sunny morning. We gather

---

[6] Doesn't she ever want to sit with anyone else?

speed at the top of the hill and I spot the nearby dump. A woman in front of me speaks loudly on her mobile: 'Oh I know. Haha. No, no. I didn't dare point it out. I'm on my way back now, hon, we're just leaving town. See if they'll keep at it.'

The crazies are on board. A stout little man stumbles over to me, his eyes scrunched so tight they look like belly buttons. 'Hey,' I say. He stammers an exhale and nods. 'You alright?' I ask. He takes my hand; I shake it and say, 'Nice to meet you.' His puts his other hand on top of mine, dry and soft like a dog's paw. When I retract my hand he keeps smiling, reaches out and cups my face. 'Alright then, come on!' someone shouts, and he retreats to his seat. One guy gives me a headache just to watch: rapidly leaning forward and backward, neck tensed against the force, shouting 'Haaangh!' every other second. His guardian smiles like there's nothing to notice. They are often on these early buses. Do they insist on coming out for a few hours in town or is it the carers' idea? Is it good for their health to leave their enclosure? We take a sharp right at the mental home, left at Roxby where the bell sounds and the driver slows us down for the stop they get off at. The woman in front of me turns her head and I see it's in fact a pencil case she's been talking into.

I park the newspaper trolley at the foot of a cracked drive, my fingertips grey and shiny with ink. My iPod plays Nine Inch Nails, who make everything feel important, even opening the flap of another letterbox and pushing a paper through that'll only get thrown straight in the bin. Rhythms on *The Downward Spiral* sound like coal-burning machinery, grime and oil boiling between pistons, spliced with skin-breaking drum hits; the guitars and synths threaten to swallow everything in erratic gales of noise.

But Trent Reznor, the lead vocalist, is *really* atheist. He must have a chip on his shoulder about religion, about God himself. The lyrics put up a wall where I can't quite relax and love the music; something about it rubs off on me like muck. A faint idea that I shouldn't be listening to it. In case I agree with him, maybe. I've even deleted their song 'Heresy' from my iTunes library because he yells "God is dead and no one cares".

Fifty or sixty papers are left in the trolley when I get home. I heave them into the recycling box in the garage, on top of last week's wad. The pile towers a foot above the box's brim. A few slide off and spill their leaflets. The company is slowly reducing my payment for this paper round, as though I won't notice, so I'm slowly delivering fewer papers.

It's only half twelve. Jordan won't be home for another three hours twenty; James, four hours fifteen; Dad, five hours; Mum, it's anyone's guess. The college bus, containing Emma, pulls into the nearest stop in four hours thirty-five. I microwave a tin of rice pudding, slop a spoonful of jam into it and tuck in. Rinse out and throw away the can, wash the bowl, remove evidence I was here in the day. Get changed and head out again, down the long hill to the gym.

Say hi to Dean the manager. Hi to the midlife who practically lives here, reading home improvement magazines on the wicker sofa area or stretching in her ochre tracksuit, flaunting the turkey baster-shaped sweat patch running up her arse crack that I wish I could stop glancing over at.

Nobody talks at dinner tonight. Yesterday's in the air still. Cutlery *dink dink dinks* and scrapes our plates. Glasses touch down on placemats with a *knock*. A sniff. James tries to make conversation. Mum, who was kept back at work until half seven, says, 'Mmhm'. I sit there with a quiet hatred of my dad that stops me looking up from my runner beans and potato croquettes. I don't know how I feel about Mum anymore. My phone buzzes in my pocket: Emma wants to come round – she's not seen me today. I ignore it. We clear the plates and wash up in silence. As soon as the last plate hits the draining board Dad exits the kitchen. A few seconds later, a door slams. Mum sits back at the table, crosses one leg over the other and looks at the wall. Her bag of work beside her chair. She's still in her coat. James says something else and then gives up and leaves.

Jordan says, 'What are you doing now?'

'Don't know,' I say, stood by the rumbling kettle.

'Can I go on Xbox?'

I make five cups of tea. Put one beside Dad in the living room, who says, 'Thank you,' and one on the table in front of Mum. Me and Jordan go upstairs. James is in his room, warming wax between his finger and thumb and twisting his hair into place.

'Cheers,' he says when I put the drink between him and the surfboard mirror.

'Where are you off?' I say.

'Gonna see if Mum will let me borrow the car to go see someone.'

At my desk I open the laptop and sign into MSN. Change my name from 322 to 321.

Up pops the conversation box from Emma – she doesn't waste a second.

Hey, it reads.

Jordan turns my Xbox on. He sits there quietly whilst I type away. Ten minutes later, he turns round and smiles. 'My guy's ace,' he says, referring to the character he's created on *Elder Scrolls: Oblivion*. 'Look.'

The conversation between me and Emma scrolls up the MSN window, our faces, on webcam, to its right. Emma's slightly pixelated face flickers blue and red from her family TV. If I don't reply for a few seconds, her eyes track to the left to watch whatever they've got on. When I hit send, her eyes return to our conversation.

She asks why I haven't been replying today, why I don't want to see her.

I say there's work to catch up on and try explaining how unwell I've felt.

it always seems to be when I want to see you that you feel poorly, Emma says.

Is that really what you think?

sometimes, I guess

I watch her straight face and can't think what to say. She starts to type again. I click off MSN and shut my laptop. In the sketchbook beside it I draw a spiral, then add spikes to its outer curve. From the speakers behind me I hear swords bashing shields, men and monsters shouting in pain, the classical soundtrack, the Xbox's fans whirring.

'Can you come off that, now?' I say to Jordan. 'You'll get it overheated.' He glances at me, turns back to the screen, then glances twice more when he notices I'm staring at him. 'Now,' I add when he doesn't save and quit straight away.

He turns the Xbox off, puts the controller on the shelf and sits back on the bed.

'No, can you just go somewhere else?'

He gets up, takes his empty mug and the American football he for some reason takes everywhere with him, heads through to his room, and leaves his door open in case I change my mind. I shut my door.

Emma sends a long text. Opens by apologising for sounding mean. Wonders why I sometimes manage, despite attending college, to avoid seeing her all day. Why I cancel everything we do and how her hopes are raised and then dashed in the process, over and over. *Is it really that hard?* she asks. What stands out is where she writes, *I'm not so much tired as I am SICK of it.* She closes it with another apology, that it's only because she misses me, etc., etc. But it's that sentence, *SICK of it*, that echoes.

Do you think I can turn it off and on? I reply. *Only feel ill when it's convenient? When it gets me out of going somewhere? Dont you think I* want *to see you?* My body trembles a little. Sweat wets my armpits. And this fucking phone can't keep up with my typing. I end the message with *Dont bother replying.*

A text comes back full of more apologies. I clap my phone shut.

Heavy rain patters on the window. I open the blinds and it looks amazing: the sun is right down in a parting between houses, lighting the downpour from behind. I take some pictures just as it thins to a shower. Then remove the memory card, put it in my laptop and start editing the pictures on Photoshop. I'm good at this. I could never afford Photoshop, but a few kind words to the Media department technician at college snagged me an illegal copy.

Jordan's footsteps pad across the landing.

'I say,' I call.

But he doesn't hear. He thunders down the stairs, the way he does. Like someone's tipped a wheelbarrow of rocks down them. I wanted to say, 'I think it's cooled down now, if you wanted to carry on.'

18

'We were waiting on the bus last night and all the Lindsey girls from school came on in those hairdressing scrubs. Black scrub things. One of them fucking stunk of fish as they walked past. I thought, *that's right, you scratty bitch*,' Ben says in the Maggy May.

'Jesus, alright.' I shade a drawing of two faceless people sat on a sofa watching a TV that's half-swallowed into the trunk of a tree.

My insides are tender: I try not to move too much. Or laugh at Ben's rants. Laughing shakes the abdomen. Keep all amusement to a big grin, or if necessary one sharp exhale through the nose: one jolt of the diaphragm. A swamp stagnates in the bowl shape of my stomach, its surface coagulating, lit by a bulb that dangles from the cesspit's fleshy ceiling.

Ben leans back and starts untangling his earphone wires. He's wearing a black *Hail to the Thief* t-shirt. He went to see Radiohead with Holly last weekend, before telling her it was a waste of a ticket to take her, that she isn't even a fan, that he should have taken me. I'm so glad he didn't ask me to go, even if it might have been the best night of my life. The journey in his stern dad's people carrier with the knob attached to the steering wheel, the rushing crowds at the show, the crush between bodies obstructing any escape. Not even Radiohead could make me go through that.

Emma comes through the big automatic doors with George, Cartwright and that friend with prominent teeth who's always here but I've never heard him speak. Emma's eyes meet mine as she gets close. She puts her arms round my middle. Rests her cheek on my shoulder, turning away from everyone else. 'Are we okay yet?' she says quietly. I put my free hand on her shoulder. She's mentioned spending some time with her dad this afternoon, before he goes to work in London. But look at this closeness with me; is it leading to an announcement that she's changed her mind, and wants to come over to mine now? You can't let me relax and then change your mind.

'Are we off then?' Ben says[7] when Holly arrives with her big smile.

'Where's Dale?' I ask.

'Dropped out completely.' Cartwright lands in a chair, takes his beanie off and throws it onto the table. 'He never went to his lessons anyway, all last term.'

'Shit,' I say, waiting for someone to ask me if that sounds familiar.

Ben picks up his bag, rolls it onto his back and holds the strap that hangs over his collarbone. 'He got kicked out, definitely.'

Emma holds my hand and doesn't say anything on the walk. Daisies have flowered around our feet in patches as big as tennis courts, stretching to the sections of park I don't know, round the back of the conifer row, over the crest of that slope. Goosebumps tighten the skin of my arms, even though it's sunny. As we pass the dried-up fountain Emma puts her other hand on top of mine for a minute. I watch the homeless guy sat on the fountain wall, chin tucked into his chest, looking at all the carrier bags he's set down.

Past the post depot, over the junction, past the big church with gravestones on the lawn. I tell Ben about my English assessments, making them sound as complicated as I can; he doesn't laugh at how simple my subjects are when Ryan's not around. Emma walks in front of us and I can't help noticing she's gained weight.

The fragile nausea I felt before ebbs away. I risk buying a steak bake and Arabian Coke.

On the bus, I finally ask Emma, 'Are you still seeing your dad?'

'Yes,' she deflates. 'Don't worry.'

It makes me mad again but I keep quiet.

The driver argues with a lad trying to get off at a stop in Winterton, then he shouts over his shoulder, down the aisle, 'You

---

[7] Leaving college early is good, but it makes me nervous to travel with friends. They can see me, they know me, they can talk about me. They are there with me on this early bus, ready to spectate an illness. Should I wait another hour so that I can travel alone? Well no, that means an extra hour at college. Anything can develop in an hour. And if I miss that next bus, the only choice will be the one with Winterton kids on it. A boiling kettle of chatter, laughter, swarming movement. And what if *they* saw me being sick?

don't just get off wherever you want. Your pass is to take you home, not to your mate's houses. I'll be checking them.'[8]

Home by two. I drag my bedroom cupboard, tall drawers, book-cases and bedside table out onto the landing. Hoover the embossed sections of dusty carpet where they were. Open the window because I'm sweating. Plan a different position for everything. It's a small space. When I'm pushing the tall drawers back in, the sides come loose and it falls apart. I put its carcass in place and bash the loose bits back together. Lean out the window for a while and wonder if I do this shit every fortnight because I'm frustrated about things that sit below my attention. Then I hoover again. Arrange the wiring of the monitor, speakers, laptop, Xbox, lamp. Polish all the surfaces.

Two little drawers slot into the bedside table. One is full of wires, adapters and instruction manuals still in their plastic packaging, the other is what Ben once coined a guy's "Drawer of Sin". The one with the condoms. Disposing of used condoms isn't as simple as putting it in my paper bin, and certainly not the kitchen bin, and if you flush them down the bog they apparently come back to haunt you. Mine wait in the Drawer of Sin. Slumped there like sad little parcels until it's safe to put them in a bag and head through the house to hide them under the trash in the dustbin, outside. But sometimes I daren't touch them: old sex residue makes me think I'll get a sickness bug if the bodily juices transfer to my mouth. So they might stay there for a few days, or a week. The bottom of the drawer has acquired a thin film of Johnny grease. At the back, where

---

[8] What? He can't do that. If I become ill and need to jump off, will he not let me? Even if I whisper to him how desperate I am? Is that just this driver, or is it a new rule they all follow? There's still the emergency lever. Surely that will open the door, no matter what the rules are. Of course it will. I'm okay now, though. Relax. And in future, the day I need to jump off, we might have a different driver, who doesn't care where I get off. Or we might have the one I had a go at, who might press a button that doesn't even let me open the doors when I pull the emergency lever thing. And I'll be at the front, ragging the lever, punching the glass, whilst vomit comes out my mouth and shit comes out the bottom of my trousers.

it's still dry, my dead grandfather's old signet ring rests on a wooden box I made at school.

When I pull open the box's lid, letters from Emma spring up and try to unfold themselves. I sit on my bed, put them down beside me and rifle through the mementos they were burying. An empty, torn-up packet of mints that I've flattened and preserved with Sellotape. A black leather bracelet, chewed out of shape. A single bark chipping. A photo of me flying above my grandparents' hedge.

She hand-writes each letter. Sneaks them into my backpack[9] or hands them over and points a finger at me, saying, 'Now don't read this until you're alone tonight.' Pages torn out of her notebook, with bits of the laddered paper still dangling off their left edges. The letters go on forever, and just when the end seems mercifully near – *Well, it's 3:05 in the morning. I really should go to sleep but I just wanted to write this since I was thinking about you. I bet you're all cute and asleep right now. I love it when we're cuddling in your bed* – off she'll go for half a dozen more pages.

What we have is so amazing, she writes.

Is it? She barely sees me once or twice a week. All I do is keep my head down and draw, feeling sick.

I feel so incredibly lucky that you're mine.

Why? I cancel on every plan either of us make.

I loved the time that [nondescript thing we did that I didn't commit to memory].

She'll inevitably refer to the time I comforted her when Perdita died, calling me her "rock", which is annoyingly dramatic. She'll write about our sex, how brilliant it is, certain moments she will never forget, and I'll feel my dick harden, remembering it. And then the letter will close with rows upon rows of kisses, and an annotation beside them telling me that the kisses equate to the exact number of days we've been going out.

---

[9] In one side pocket are all my tablets for emergency illness, which I worry Emma might discover during her letter-sneaking. How I'll shrink if she asks me what they're for.

And I'll reply. It really makes her day when she gets a letter back. I comment on how unexpected and wonderful a surprise her letter was. Apologise that it's taken me a while to write. Agree about how great everything is between us. Circumnavigate the things she wrote about wanting to be with me forever, maybe put a few more compliments instead. Do a paragraph or two of erotica. Then I get ready for the marathon of trying to at least match the number of kisses she writes.

If not a full letter, it's a little note she wrote whilst thinking about me in class. Or it's a long text. A quick sentence, a line of kisses, a little essay. After an argument, after a perfect night.

'Here,' I say on the bus one bright, wet morning, opening my bag.

'Or there,' Emma replies, then laughs when I frown up at her whilst rummaging.

My fingers find the folded wad of paper. 'My reply to the other day. Now, listen. You're not to open it until you get home. See, it says it there.' I put it in her hands, pointing to the instructions I've written on the cover. 'Stop feeling it. There's no money inside.'

'Nor a ring? I'm kidding.'

'Are you?'

The dirt road widens and we slow beneath the gardens in Winteringham.

'Here comes your girlfriend,' Emma says.

Skull Lady holds her arm out to hail the bus. Either she's purposefully doing a stiff-armed wave or she can't keep it still. It goes up and down like a seismograph needle on a quiet day.

'Shit, you'd better scarper,' I say. Even as we joke, I feel bad.

The bus pulls over. A transparent hood with butterflies on it shelters Skull Lady's white perm from the spits of rain. The doors open and she climbs the two steps aboard. She stands by the driver. Her thumb and fingers pinch the flap of her coat pocket, as though testing its texture. She pulls but the two pocket buttons don't open. The hem of her coat just tugs up an inch. Instead of trying again she curls her hand under the flap and squeezes it between the buttons, and those startling wrist bones show. She pulls out her bus pass. It's in a clear zip-lock sandwich bag. To save it getting wet. Even though it's laminated. It's almost too sad to bear. She holds it out to the driver, her hand moving about as though writing on a whiteboard.

'It's like when you've got a fake ID and you don't want the bouncer to know you're only fourteen, so you wave it about like fuck to stop him reading it properly.'

Emma laughs. 'You love her.'

'Only for that body she's rocking.'

'Oh God.'

'She'll have a few men on the side in Scunny. That's why she gets on every morning. Her husband thinks she's playing pontoon with her friends when she's actually getting spit-roasted by two other blokes.'

Emma pinches me and says '*Shhh*!' and we giggle.

We're eight or nine rows back but no one at the front's giving their seat up so I stand and gesture Skull Lady to mine. I go hold onto one of the bars near the driver.

My phone buzzes.

Thanks!lolxxxxxxxxxxxxx

Emma's smiling at me. I write back.

its me who had 2 scarper lol xxxxxx

Your 2 favourite girls sat togetherxxxx

Why does Skull Lady really get on the bus every morning, when clearly it almost kills her? Why leave home so early every day at that age? Doesn't she have a relative to take her by car? Where does she go when she gets off in town? Is it something she *has* to do? Does she do it for herself or through devotion to someone else?

Me and Emma glance at each other and smile all the way to college. At one point I look over and she doesn't notice. She's looking out the window, her hands on top of the folders on her lap, and she looks amazing. Yes, I do love her.

19

'We've gone,' Dad shouts up the stairs – the first sentence directly steered towards me since the university evening.

My family are off to watch Man-United play at Old Trafford.

A few nights before the match, I told Mum I couldn't go, expecting another row, but she said 'Okay.' Dad found out and said nothing.

'How come you aren't coming?' Jordan asked a few minutes ago, as they were getting ready to leave.

'Don't fancy it,' I lied. I know how long it takes to get to Manchester. The distance, the stuffy car, the dense traffic clotting the motorway. And I can't do it.

The front door shuts.

I sit for a long time doing nothing at all.

20

Ben invites us all round his on a Friday night, but I'm too nervous to go. It's the first time I've backed out of something taking place so close by – barely a ten-minute walk away. Emma's going there. That's why. I can't disappear if I'm ill without her following me home, without then untangling myself from her, having to be subtle, waiting until it would no longer seem rude to ask when she's leaving, whilst inwardly screaming to be alone.

At about half nine there's a knock at the front door that I recognise and my insides fall to bits. I come downstairs and see the wobbly little portrait through the obscured glass. Open the door to Emma's big smile.

'Thought I'd leave early and surprise you,' she says.

She sees my face. It sticks a pin into her happy expression. I stand back from the door to let her in. She lowers her head and goes past me.

I sit at the kitchen table and she sits adjacent to me.

'I walked up with Ryan, as far as his house. There wasn't much going on at Ben's. It wasn't the same without you there. Got to snaffle some cheesy chips off Holly, though. Just thought I'd come here for a bit.'

I don't reply.

'Didn't you want me to come?'

I shake my head. It's very hard to talk. Sickness licks up my stomach. There's an aching spin behind my eyes. Beads of tree sap form down the walls of my throat, sticking it together when I swallow. How could she just show up? The one place I feel safe in this world and she breaks in to *surprise me*.

Emma falls quiet. She looks around, palms together between her thighs.

'I thought you might be happy I came to see you.'

I put my two thumbnails together and press them so that the skin beneath them goes pale. Bite off the skin beside the nail. Twist my fingers to make the joints click.

'I'll text Mum,' Emma says. I nod and watch her do it. Wait for the reply. 'She says she'll be ten minutes. She's just finishing her tea.'

I do a big exhale with inflated cheeks and don't say another word whilst we wait.

Jordan comes in to get a drink and sees us. His eyebrows pinch together, his mouth turns down, bottom lip rolled out.

'Am I interrupting something?'

He pours himself some milk, takes a bag of Doritos from the cupboard and leaves.

'I shouldn't have come,' Emma says to the table.

I watch the oven clock blink away five slow, silent minutes. I manage to run my fingers over Emma's hand, because a normal person wouldn't be furious. She's tried to be impulsive and nice; I want her to know I don't hate her. She looks up at me but I focus on her hand. How the soft skin gathered at her knuckles moves a little with my sweeping fingers, and I can feel the bone.

After she leaves, I send a text. *I need you to promise me something xx*
Sure, what?xxxxx
That you'll never come round again without me saying that you can x

21

Horkstow Road is one of the poshest stretches of Barton. Long and straight: the south edge of town. Fields on one side, swanky houses on the other, set way back behind low walls, perfect lawns and rock formations lit by spotlights when it's night.

A massive old tree, whose dead spouse lies beside it in neatly sawn but left-to-rot pieces, marks the entrance to a farmer's track that cuts between two wheat hills, away from the big houses, away from town. We used to stand down here, my friends and me, and watch the fireworks on bonfire night shoot up from the park half a mile away. I would have a bottle of ale on the floor beside me and my arms around a girl I fancied, hands warming in her hoodie pocket.

I check the time on my phone: English Language is in session, way over there in Scunthorpe. I can scarcely picture my empty seat.

The nausea that woke up with me has faded, now I'm away.

Then get on the next bus and go to the afternoon lessons, at least.

No, it's too far. Too *observed*. A trap.

If I could only teleport into my seat and know I could vanish again. Can't there be a way to shrink the distance? Can't these fields just be erased in the night, when no one's looking?

At the end of the farmer's track is a bramble-tangled slope way up to the dual carriageway above. Ben took a picture of me throwing a chair from the top a few weeks ago, captioned it "Ancient Bartonian hunting method". I remember where it landed and clamber up to fish it out of the weeds. A little red metal chair with two wooden circles, one to support your back, the other to place your arse. It's wet and rotting. Thin partings have opened in the grain and house teal fungus crumbs, like deposits of dried toothpaste. I don't want to sit on it; the dirty moisture will transfer into my jeans, onto my skin. But what else is there to do? Whether I sit on it or not, will I *ever* make it to college again? I think about the coming exams: three hours, three times. Deadly silence.

In this overgrown corner of the field where the ploughs don't reach, I dot the chair around, looking for level ground, sit down.

The thin legs pierce the soil and I sink until the wooden seat meets the grass, my own legs stretched out in front of me so they don't get trapped beneath it.

It'll be a few hours before I can safely return home: Mum's not at work today. If I can make it until after lunch, I can at least say I didn't have lessons in the afternoon and she should believe me. I rest my bag on my shins, select Radiohead on my iPod and begin listening through all of their albums.

Once bored of sitting in the grass, I pace about. The pace settles into a straight line that I walk along, turn, go the other way, turn, come back. I keep the walk slow to stop any false sense of time passing quicker than it is, of distance being covered, of progress being made. By the time *The Bends* finishes and I play *OK Computer*, I notice the line I'm walking is becoming visible. The trodden, damaged grass is darker than the rest.

Throughout *Kid A*, I watch the sunken chair go past me on the right, turn and watch it go past me on the left. The weather doesn't change. It's like there is no weather. I go through phases of walking faster, walking with heavier feet, stomping a path. I play *Amnesiac* and walk slower for a while.

Midday. Mum wouldn't buy it if I went home this early, but look: someone's coming, round the long bend of the field. A big black dog runs in front of him, fetching an item he then throws for it again. I don't need to explain why I'm not at college to a stranger, but could I explain what I'm doing here, full stop? I spare a last look at the faint brown path I've trod over the last four hours, and set off back up the farmer's track, towards the dog walker and Barton behind him.

As we get closer I see the dog walker is Bitty's dad. Bitty is an old friend I've known through primary and secondary school. I went to his house as a child and played *Goldeneye 64* with him after school and never dared use his toilet for the piss I painfully needed. He had a massive rabbit in a tiny cage and his dad entered garden competitions so we couldn't touch the lawn. He had a sister with leukaemia whose hair was thin and voice trembled. As a group of mates, we weren't very nice to Bitty throughout secondary school, despite him being nice. Jokes just seemed to come easy. His closeness to his mum brought up weird comments about "family bath time". Puberty gave Bitty a miss. We hounded him about his dad, whose nasal voice, rosy cheeks and Roman nose earned him the name Nige, short for Nigel Thornberry, the cartoon character. We'd do impressions of him in front of Bitty. And just when ammunition ran dry, we found out Nige's job was some kind of tax collector, which kept us going for another year. Bitty developed a tough skin, but I still regret it. I never joined in quite like others, but my hands aren't clean, and I got a lot of shit through school too, so I should've known better. We still see him sometimes. A few months ago his sister passed away, only weeks after learning the cancer was back.

I try to look confident when saying hi to Nige as we pass each other, as though it's perfectly normal that I'm down here alone with my college bag. He says hi back, gives off a hint of confusion. Or suspicion. I put my earphone back in and carry on listening to *Hail to the Thief*.

22

Emma follows me out of the rain, into clothes shops for her and music shops for me. We wait in town for the bus back to Barton, holding hands and laughing about things I'll never remember. Despite our best efforts, we're soon soaked. Emma's hair bunches together like dark rope and I taste hair product that's dribbled down my face. We jump on the 350 and although May fast approaches, we both shiver and cling to each other for warmth all the way to my house.

Emma pokes fun at me for wanting to dry her hair. The sound of a hairdryer, or any loud fan, is massively comforting. In Art class, people use hairdryers to quickly set a layer of paint before applying the next one, and as soon as one turns on I'll want to fall asleep. At home, I use a dilapidated orange thing from the 80s that Mum used to own; it's old, loud, and takes ages to dry anything – that's why I use it.

I set some of my lounge bottoms and a t-shirt out for Emma and help her peel off her clothes. But as soon as I see her pale wet skin I get wildly turned on and pull her on top of me, kissing, biting, sucking, grabbing handfuls of her. She goes straight for my belt; I hear a rip when I'm taking my top off, frustrated at it clinging to me. Our skin is cold from the rain; the heat I feel enclose me when I put myself inside her makes me throb and throb. Her wet hair trails all over my face and I laugh.

We spend the rest of the day in pyjamas. I mention needing to do work. Laying the foundations down, you know, in case I suddenly need her to leave. But five o'clock passes and I still feel alright, and I know her mum's finished work now so Emma has a lift at the ready, which makes me all the more comfortable and even happy with her being here. My brothers and parents arrive and we order Chinese food.

* * *

My Art teacher has a face like Rowan Atkinson having an allergic reaction; his toothpick frame is bandaged in black clothes. He speaks quietly with his arse-shaped chin aloft, mincing between the tables, before invariably announcing, 'I'm just going for a quick wee,' every lesson. Why does he have to say "wee"? It makes me picture it streaming out, pungent and dark.

The class has gone to the local art gallery. Our parents had to fill a form to give us permission to go, and mine never saw it.

'We could catch up with them in my car,' Rowan Atkinson says in the vacant classroom. He does a weak smile. 'I'm willing to break the rules if you are.'

This wasn't part of the plan.

I exchange a glance with the girl who forgot to bring her permission form in. She shrugs.

'Don't worry about it,' I say to the teacher. 'I don't want you to get in trouble for my sake.'

Sat at the high table in the Maggy May, I concentrate on not being sick. My insides are too ripe; my stomach's going sweet and rotten, fermenting; its softening flesh secretes sweet juices that I taste when I burp. The lessons I'm meant to be in slug by. People speak to me but I can't open my mouth. Emma puts a hand under my arm and her head on my shoulder. She finds my hand and strokes the top of it, over the veins, the knuckles, down the fingers, again and again, content not to talk, my hands dry and rough, hers soft. She does this for an hour without a word.

'Got to go,' she then says. Squeezes my hand and disappears.

I draw little patterns in the margin of my notebook. Every movement I make, even breathing, wakes the urge to vomit.

I harass Mum with texts until she agrees to come and pick me up. It's her day off. I imagine what she will be doing before she sets off – gathering her handbag, putting her shoes on, locking the front door behind her, giving the car a second to warm up whilst unfolding the glasses she keeps on the dashboard – and add this to the time it takes to get from home to college, taking into account her cautious driving, to work out how long I'll have to wait.

When she arrives, I stand up real slow; my stomach will slosh liquid with too sudden a movement. Luckily none of my friends are here to see this.

Mum's not impressed.

'Thanks for coming,' I say. And then, 'Sorry you had to come.'

We're in the college car park. There's a bunch of cars blocking the way round to the exit so Mum turns, reverses, turns, reverses, to get us facing the way she came in. 'For *God's* sake,' she says, craning to see over her bumper.

Students walk about between the cars, across the sports fields, up and down the paths.

We pull onto the main road and a horrible thought crosses my mind: what if Mum doesn't take me home? What if she just drives in the opposite direction? She might say: 'It's time you got over this *thing* of yours. We're going far away. It's for your own good.' She's done it before. So to speak. Driving further and further when I begged her to take me home. Fuck's sake. Is there *no* reliable escape home? Buses break down, arrive late or not at all. Mum's usually at work, and look at how long it's taken for her to come get me when she isn't. Dad's out of the question. James has passed his test but doesn't have a car.

I *am* ill this time, I'm sure of it. I wasn't just worried.

Yet even as we're driving, getting closer to Barton by the second, I feel the nausea starting to ebb. *Why?* I wish it would stay, just to know it was real. The *intense* sickness I felt all day at college was *real*. As bad as the day in Kennedy Space Center last summer, which similarly fizzled away after I took those painkillers. Do I have a condition where sickness starts and stops this quickly? Mum doesn't talk all the way home.

A couple of hours later I slip out and go to meet Ant at the gym. I know Mum will resent me all the more, but I have to go. If I don't work out at least every other day, it's like I can feel myself shrinking. If I miss two days in a row, I look in the mirror and wonder if I can see the muscle loss. I know it's stupid. But a few more bicep curls won't hurt anyone.

'You know what's proper weird,' Ant says, putting two twenty-two-point-fives back on the rack and sitting on the end of a bench. 'When you're getting head but you need a piss. It's like: it's so good, but you don't feel sure she won't... suck it out of you. And sometimes I think it's even better than getting head when you *don't* need a piss. But there's a risk. It's like: this is nice, but am I pissing?' His deadly serious, pensive face cracks a massive grin when I start laughing.

23

Emma yelps, covers her face and runs into me when a pigeon flaps right past us. 'Fucking pigeons!' she says.

'It wouldn't have flown into you.'

'You don't know that! They barely know how to fly. They're like drunk flyers. They're evil. Look at them!' A gang of pigeons scuttle across the block-paved road in front of our feet, doing indecisive little flaps. Emma shudders.

Sebastian, happy to remain quiet, has that sort of bob in his walk that only seriously tall people can have. He smiles at what we're saying, then he frowns to himself, working out a thought or visiting a memory.

'A bird's flown into me before,' I say. 'I was walking down to Ben's in, like, Year Ten, and I plucked a leaf off a hedge beside the path, and this fucking bird shot out and hit me here.' I touch my temple. 'It caned. I think its beak jabbed in.'

Emma laughs – that choking giggle. 'You're not helping.'

This is amazing. Emma's coming home with me and the nausea is barely there.

'Shall we go in here?' I say beside a Costa. 'I could go for a coffee. We've got just over quarter of an hour.'

'Sure.' Sebastian's eyebrows go up, happy to be woken from his daydream.

I order a latte. Emma and Sebastian get hot chocolate. We find some sofas by the window and sit down. 'Look at us, all sophisticated,' Emma says, stirring her drink. She takes a sip, then looks up at me with pursed lips, ready to laugh: there's a dab of cream on the end of her nose. Hilarious, I think, doing a smile and listening to her giggle.

Two thirds into the journey home my guts clench and gurgle.

Oh no. Has the latte disagreed with me?

I'm sat next to Emma, a panic coming over me.

My stomach cramps again, like my body is trying to shit without me having any control over it. Another cramp. My guts are being wrung like a wet rag.

Hold it together.

I'm going to shit my pants. Right here. In front of Emma and Sebastian and all the seniors riding the bus at this time.

We're in Winteringham, where I'd normally start feeling safe. But I need to be home *right fucking now*. What the fuck's happening?

Help me, God. Please. Shall I take an Imodium tablet? No, it takes an hour to work, according to the packet, and that's not quick enough. And taking a tablet is admitting that I've got diarrhoea and this is a catastrophe.

The bus stops.

A man gets on and pushes coins under the glass to the driver.

A man gets on and shows a bus pass.

A woman pays, steps back off the bus, re-appears with one of those trolleys old people push about, heaves it on board, slowly wheels it round so she can push it along to her seat.

The doors shut, the engine blows a gale and we crawl away. Out the village, along the tight bumpy roads, then back onto the main stretch to Ferriby. I brace myself for another squeeze. It lasts a lifetime. My insides are hot. I look over at Sebastian and everyone else sat lifelessly bored, jostled about by the road.

'I can't have you round today,' I mumble.

Emma lifts her hands up a few inches and lets them flop down onto her lap.

'*Why?*'

'I don't feel so good.'

'You *always* say that. I've got nowhere to go.' Day buses only go as far as Barton, not the next village, where she lives. 'I'll have to go to the doctor's and wait for Mum to finish work. And that will be over three hours.'

Staring down at the seat in front, I don't know what to say.

Thank God her mum's working at the surgery today.

The bus pulls into my stop. Can I make the minute-long walk between here and home?

'Sorry,' I say, and get up.

Mum's car is on the drive; I can hear the hoover whilst I'm unlocking the front door.

'Thank you,' I say under my breath to God, heading inside.

The hurt text from Emma will come soon. She'll be writing it now. I'll keep texting her whilst she's waiting at the surgery. I am the worst boyfriend.

I don't even go to the bathroom.

24

Spending time with Emma on a weekend becomes too hard, unless it's to see other people as well. Having others around dilutes the focus she'll have on me, even if it means being in the sight of more people. The scrutiny should be less. And it means I could retreat without Emma being left completely alone. On college nights, I have the excuse of needing to hit the hay at a good time ready for the next early morning, or that I'd better get on with some work. Weekend days are big expanses of time; there's no reason to wait till the evening to see each other, no reason not to stay up late or stop over.

How do I occupy the days so that I can say I'm too busy?

How do I put a cap on how long we see each other?

In the week days, we talk about her coming over for a few hours, but then I cancel at least half the time.

'Are you getting tired of me?' Emma asks on a sunny ride home when I wriggle out of seeing her.

'No.'

Or maybe I am.

I don't cancel on a whim. It's because the closer it gets to her coming over or me going to her place, the more the sickness grips my neck and foams in my stomach, until it's too much to bear and I **know** I'll be sick in front of her.

Most days, I'm already at home when the bus comes in from Leggott, and I send a desperate *Don't come tonight xx* text with barely a minute to spare. One evening, she's already got off the bus at my stop, and has to wait by the road for a lift home. I'm sat on the floor of my bedroom gripping my hair and waiting for my phone to buzz with verbal abuse. But Emma's not like that. She'll show exasperation, but will never punish. Maybe I just don't let her. My ace in the hole with every would-be argument is that these stakes aren't as high for me. I don't care if it results in breaking up. I don't need her. Without her around **watching me** I wouldn't worry about being sick so often. College would be easier. I could see my friends without the slow turning in my stomach. People would remember that I'm a lone wolf. So I push harder, be mean; she'll submit because our relationship is more important than winning a fight.

But I still cower inside when I hit send on another text letting her down.

It's a Saturday night and I cave at the last minute.

Are you sure? We're in the car!xxxxx she replies.

Is she now sat there with her mum, waiting to hear from me if they should start the engine? I think how embarrassing this would be for me, were the shoe on the other foot.

She's round my house one night after I cancel and then re-invite her.

'But not today!' Emma says, in a kind of teacherly voice, when one of us mention something to do with sex.

'I know why you're doing that,' I say. 'Playing that "you can't have sex with me" game, as though depriving me would teach me a lesson or something. Or keep me under control. I don't even want to have sex. You watch too much TV.'

We've been together six months now and we haven't spent one whole night together. This is my fault.

When Emma comes over, we cuddle, have various forms of sex, and then I wait the appropriate amount of time before asking when she's getting picked up. She's learned the routine. She sighs, part serious, part joking, texts her mum, receives the reply and says, 'Mum's coming in an hour,' her phone screen lighting up her face. I count the minutes, nausea growing, convinced that *tonight is the night* a sickness bug takes hold. She makes hints: a yawn and mention of how sleepy she is when it gets to eleven or so at night. Sometimes we start drifting to sleep, before I feel like I can't go any further; I squeeze her awake and ask when she's leaving. Her mum comes to get her even if it's gone one in the morning.

When I go round to Emma's house, I already have an escape plan ready for a couple of hours later. Emma, whether we're alone or in front of her family, will clutch onto me and say, 'Nope, I'm not letting you go!' and I entertain her for a minute before pulling myself up and shaking her off, smiling to her dad.

After a couple more rejections, her family seem to get the idea that I'm never going on any day trips with them, and give up. But once a month, they go to see the extended family in London, and Emma's started inviting me. 'Everyone always asks about you. I want to show you off,' she says. But I don't go. I get smacked with images of being squished in their family car for the five-hour ride down there, trying to breathe, having to be polite to her relatives, sleeping on the floor of her nanna's house. Wanting to leave in the night. Having nowhere to escape to. Running out onto the dark streets and looking for a place to hide.

So we do little else but sit in Emma's living room, watching footy on the TV. I turn down cups of tea. Then I go home, feeling like I've defied death.

Emma and me are lying in bed when I learn her older sister Miranda doesn't like me, no doubt because she sees the tears when I cancel on Emma one time too many.

'You might as well tell me what she said.'

'It's honestly nothing. I shouldn't have mentioned it.'

I don't reply, and the silence makes Emma carry on.

'She doesn't think you treat me very well. Sometimes. She says I could do better.'

We stay still. The words worm in and make me furious. I want to take my arm from under Emma.

'Sorry,' Emma says. 'It's not what I think. Are you alright?'

It takes a long time to gather an answer. 'Well not really. That's, like, one of the worst things I've heard said about me, behind my back.'

'I think you treat me well.'

I put my clothes on and shut the bedroom door behind me. Go downstairs and sit in the kitchen. When I go back up, Emma's still in my bed, leant up on an elbow, scoring a thumb under her eyes.

25

'*Much Ado About* Fuck All,' I sigh and slap my books on the desk. Take a Polo out my pocket, nip it between my front teeth and sit down in the yellow-walled Literature room.

'Christ, Chris is in a good mood,' Keith laughs. I see our teacher watching me and realise I was louder than I meant to be.

And I laugh too. I am in a good mood.[10] It's raining outside. It's a little bit darker than usual.

The blinds are stirred by a patchy breeze; the teacher shuts the big metal windows[11] whilst talking about deception.

'Doing one of your little cross-hatches?' Laura says halfway though the lesson as I draw in the margins of my notebook. 'A tree! It's always a tree.' She leans past my arm and flicks backwards through my book. 'Tree, tree, blobby things, a candle, spikes, a tree!'

'They're fun to draw.' I smile. 'But I never finish them. The branches just split into smaller and smaller branches, and I never know when to stop.'

---

[10] 'Talk' by Coldplay blares in my head, louder than real life. The song I heard floating out the momentarily open door of Tommy's garden bar last year, after I'd necked that Famous Grouse and was sat forward on a wooden trestle in the garden, vomiting onto the black grass below me, trying to shove a fat Corgi who was eating my sick out the way with my feet, then I threw up on the dog and its stumpy tail wagged. The song repeats now: "Or *do*... something that's *never* been done." Nightmarish, delirious. Like it might make me sick. Like it connects me through time to that moment of vomiting. Causing history to repeat itself. Is it a subconscious warning? Does my body know an infection is brewing and this is how it's communicating? God, it's deafening. I should go home. Quickly, before the illness strikes.

[11] An exit is taken away. It's not like I could've jumped out the open window if I needed to escape, but look at how many people I'd have to squeeze past to get out of here through the door. Or I could vault over this table, and the table opposite me, probably slipping on the paperwork of the girls sat there. Everyone would look; the class would stop. They would remember. Especially if I'm being sick as this happens. Then there are two doors until I'm outside, into the air and the rain. But then what?

Next period, I'm sat alone at a high table in the Maggy May, drawing in the sketchbook I made with punched watercolour paper and string. It's nearly full, now. The idea is to stick these pages into my Art submission portfolio and write something about each biro drawing to make it all seem like a project. They'll see I've been doing *something* whilst not in their lessons. I got a D in the Easter assessment; the teacher wrote "Is this all you've done all year?!" in the corner of a page.

Innumerable little upward biro strokes slowly add grass on top of a rocky plateau. But it doesn't distract me from my insides, from working out travel and distance times, checking the faraway clock on the purple wall to see whether I've got time to make it into town for the next bus. I sigh and sit back, suddenly aware of the light, the day. A group of lads make a human pyramid on hands and knees near the stairs, five at the bottom, then four, three, two; a slight friend starts climbing up to be the peak and they all shout at him to hurry, then the pyramid collapses. Outside the wall of windows beside me, the rain's cleared. Smokers gather beneath the shelter down by the pond. I find *The Fellowship of the Ring* in my bag and try reading it for a while.

A girl from another table breaks off from her friends, comes over and talks to me. She's good looking, uniquely so, with a strange rosy pattern of what must be birthmarks on the left side of her face. She asks me about the book and says she takes Literature, too. In fact, we have the same teacher, just in different lessons. She talks about this, then asks where I travel in from, etc., etc. Eventually she leaves, saying she hopes to see me around.

'You were being hit on. Chris was being hit on,' Ryan says once he, Emma and a few others arrive back from Psychology and I tell them about the odd encounter.

'Balls was I. She probably just felt sorry for me sitting here reading *Lord of the* fucking *Rings*.'

But I think of how the girl's hands fidgeted with each other in front of her, how she didn't sit down.

I look at Emma, holding her big Psychology binder to her torso.

'Watch out, Emma,' Ryan says. 'Bit of friendly competition. Is she still in here?' He looks around.

'Back in a tick,' Emma says.

'I shouldn't have said anything,' I tell Ryan, watching Emma leave the Maggy May. I go after her. She potters all the way to the smaller canteen, with no idea I'm ten steps behind. She never comes in here – 'All the Scene Girls glare at me,' she says – but today, she ignores the side-on glances and finds a table. I catch up and sit beside her. Sure enough, she's sniffing and running her sleeve under her eyes. 'What's wrong?' I ask, looking at the way a teardrop can suspend between two mascaraed eyelashes. 'Honestly, I think she just felt sorry for me.'

Emma's mouth smiles without her lips parting. 'I doubt it,' she says. Sniffs, dabs eyes.

'You've got nothing to worry about. Even if she *was* interested in me, I wasn't in her. Or in anyone.' I put an arm round her.

'It's not you I'm worried about. It's other girls.'

Christ, these "other girls" again. Emma often asks if I'm sure I don't still like George. Or why I've chosen *her*, when I know girls like Sophia. She's probed about the classmate she saw me leave Literature with. She found the lipstick kiss a girl planted in my Language notebook, who kept squeezing my bicep and I didn't know how to make her stop. Emma often wonders out loud if "some good-looking girl" will swoop me away from her, as though our relationship is on borrowed time. And she *still* repeats that joke I made last autumn:

'Because I'm a nobody?'

26

The bus pulls up on a mizzly morning. I get onboard, glance at the throng of passengers and hold onto the railing. The roundabout and Top Field are pulled away from me as we accelerate away; the distance home is growing by the second. And if I get off, I'm stranded. Yes, it's a broken record.

My phone buzzes. A text from Emma – *Im upstairs! saved u a seat xxxx* – which makes me consider staying down here and later saying, 'Ah shit, I never saw your text,' once she sees me at college, but I think better of it and climb the wet helix stairs to join her.

Rattling through Scunthorpe, the urge to retch grips my throat; my diaphragm trembles and prepares to bounce my stomach contents up. Keep it together. Keep it all down. I try to focus on what I can see through the misted windows: brake lights and shop fronts. I watch a droplet of water snake down the pane, cutting a path through the mist, gathering other droplets as it goes. But it's no use. Emma's hand squeezes mine and I don't respond. If I move, I'll vomit. At the front, Sophia and her friends sit with their feet resting on the railing below the big window. Above the noise of the engine, they sing 'Umbrella' by Rihanna, emphasizing the "eh, eh, eh" bit from the chorus and laughing. So many voices up here, so much volume.

I spend ten minutes in the Maggy May, then march through the park to catch an early bus. By eleven I'm in Barton again. The weather's clear and warm now, as though college is simply a darker place than here. Down the farmer's track, the little path I worked into the clumpy grass has already gone. I sit on the bank for an hour. Listen through *With Teeth* and *The Downward Spiral* on my iPod on the walk back. Buy some chocolate and a big Relentless energy drink at the local Spar shop. Head to the gym, where Dean the manager frowns and delicately asks, 'That's… not beer, is it?'

The can of Relentless goes beside my weight bench, which I set to the declined position. I take two dumbbells from the rack and waddle back to the bench, sit with them on my knees, then in one motion lie back whilst pushing the weights up above my chest, arms outstretched. Begin pressing, down, up, down, up. The chocolate and energy drink, they swill together in my stomach as I work, but it's okay: I'm not at college. I'm not at college.

27

Do I feel sick because I'm thinking about it, or because subconsciously my brain detected a sickness I was feeling?

28

Emails about poor attendance litter my inbox. My parents aren't aware of how bad it is; at least, when Mum or Dad come home early and question why I'm there, they don't know that I probably didn't go into college at all. Mum scolds me for ages; Dad sighs and walks off. He doesn't talk directly to me anymore. In the lounge, Mum demands to know why I never stay the whole day at college, whilst Dad stares at the TV, sat very deliberately on the armchair like he's at a furniture store testing it out. If it's after dinner I'm getting bollocked, he stands over by the sink, washing up, as though he isn't listening. Then he sighs, scrunches his wet hands in a tea towel and chucks it on the side, leaves the room, and then, wait for it, a door will close. Not quite a slam, but enough force to know it was meant for me. Even Mum stops what she's saying during this short display, aware of the small chance he'll really blow up.

Since I was twelve he's gone through massive stretches of being *off* with me. For weeks at a time I would try to talk to him, and he would say 'Mm hm' without looking my way, or say nothing at all. No eye contact. He wasn't ignoring me: it was a message. I was doing something wrong.

Sigh. Walk off. Sigh.

Year Nine of school was the first time I failed to win the cross-country. Three months of sleepless nights in anticipation for the race led to disappointment: I was in the lead until halfway round and then suddenly threw up beside a flag whilst half the year group overtook me. I carried on running and still finished in the top twenty. 'You don't care anymore, do you?' Dad said that evening. And I was too angry to reply; my words congested like a sock was stuffed down my throat. Nearly a year of not speaking stretched between us. Every night brought the sighs, the sound of closing doors. I kept my head down, hating him but wishing he would talk to me. Any exchange of words was purely business: excuse me, hi, Mum's shouting you, I'm off out, pass the vinegar please, I'm home. His birthday came and went. The present and card I'd got him stayed shut in a drawer in my bedroom. 'Happy Father's Day,' I mumbled one morning the following summer as I left the bathroom and he went in. 'Thank you,' he mumbled back. It was the first we'd spoken in days. A small collection of cards accumulated in my drawer.

Now I'm sixteen, I don't want him to know his sighs work under my skin. And more than anything, I'm scared that if I spend too much time near him, I'll end up being the same.

29

Jordan makes his breakfast. Two slices of bread – toasted, buttered, jam and peanut butter plastered onto one slice, Bovril beef extract smeared onto the other, then both slices pressed together into a crispy sandwich. Six chocolate digestives. A pint-sized mug he bought from Animal Kingdom, full of strong coffee. He watches twenty-minute chunks of a film each morning, and I'll join him with my cup of tea. We don't say much. He likes to keep his morning routine undisturbed before he walks off to school.

I ask Jordan which way he takes.

'Normally meet everyone at the bottom of Forkdale and go up Stivvy, down Horkstow, then through the park, past the pool,' he says in the time it takes to dunk a wad of four biscuits into his coffee and hold them up to drip. He piles them into his mouth. 'But sometimes we go straight down Millfields. Why?'

'Just curious.'

Despite planning my walks to avoid his route, I cross paths with him a couple weeks later. My legs turn a bit jellified when I see him and his clique of mates. I've been caught. I stick my middle finger up at him as the gap closes between us and I take an earphone out, grinning.

'Alright.'

'What're you doing?' he asks.

'Working.'

His face scrunches with a smile but also suspicion, confusion. I don't look at his friends. Before Jordan has the chance to slow, I just walk through them and put my earphone back in. I walk south, out of Barton, towards Brigg. Take a left through a gap in the hedgerow. My heart settles back down, my cheeks stop burning. I hope, if he asks me about it tonight, that my parents aren't near.

Where *can* I walk? Dad works in Barton and frequently buzzes around, Nanna drives everywhere, Jordan walks to school, clearly not always on the route he told me, Emma's mum works here, my friends' parents work there, my primary school headmistress sees me every time I walk down one road, and she talks regularly to Mum. Too many people know me. They are guards, patrolling the prison camp. Or watching me from their front rooms. Everyone communicates.

'I saw Chris the other day. Down my end at, well, must have been only eight in the morning, with his backpack. I thought he goes to college at that time?'

'Yes, I *thought* he does, too…'

Eyes. Eyes.

This is why I stick to the woods and the fields. But you must cross roads to get out of Barton.

I should dig tunnels.

And even once I'm out of town, who knows who might see me? Could someone coming over the Humber Bridge see a gangly-shaped speck walking between the ponds and recognise my posture? Could Nigel and his black Labrador pass me again? I dream of a vault or panic room no one knows about but me. Or a global catastrophe, where I'm the only survivor.

30

I live in fear that Emma, in a swell of brave treachery, will show up unannounced again. Especially when I'm at home and know the Leggott bus, containing Emma, is about to pass through Barton. One night, I get a gut feeling that she's about to get off at my stop and send her a text to make sure she wasn't thinking of it.

31

Emma turns seventeen. I fill a card with an essay that bends round the printed birthday greeting. Buy a Foo Fighters CD and earrings, and wrap the little box it's presented in.

We sit in her living room, which is draped with crepe paper and balloons. 'Is this something my family will want to see?' she jokes, holding up the wrapped box, and all her family laugh.

Emma unwraps the presents, places the card open on her lap and hunches over it. This is how she always reads, and I guess that's cute. She leans on me when she gets to a nice part. Then she finishes and gives me a long kiss, which I'm used to accepting in front of her family nowadays.

'He must've put something good,' Emma's dad pretend-mumbles. 'Aren't you telling us what it says?' He grins and Emma's mum crosses her arms and kind of shuffles them left and right with a big smile.

'It's all so nice.' Emma lays an arm across me and rests her cheek on my shoulder.

But whilst I'm smiling and saying 'You're welcome' I'm busy doing mental maths: I've been here **twenty-five minutes**. If I stay for another twenty-five, that's **fifty minutes**. Each exam next week will be **three hours**. Seven twenty-five minutes fit into three hours. Imagine going through this **seven times** and there it is. That's not so bad, surely. Time may go quicker when concentrating in the exam.

Or will it slow right down? If I fell ill now, could I hold myself together for this amount of time, multiplied by seven?

Emma's mum offers me a cup of tea and I turn it down for the hundredth time. One day I'll have to accept. And accept the invitations to have dinner with them, or go on a day out, or down south to see their extended family. But not just now, thanks.

James picks me up in Mum's car, playing a CD called *Feel the Illinoise*. I comment that it sounds like something from an old-fashioned children's programme. He tells me about the party he went to last weekend. His new girlfriend's ex, Whittaker, was there, who's supposedly nuts, and the whole evening was spent keeping the fact that she's now with James hushed, lest he "go psycho".

We arrive home. James sits on the kitchen counter and I sit on a chair with my feet on the table. 'I even spoke to Whittaker every now and then, and he was alright enough, since he didn't know I was Bella's new boyfriend. But he was sniffing us all out. Like he knew it was one of us,' James carries on. 'Which made everyone else tense. He wasn't invited, but no one dared make him leave, with him being massive and like twenty-something. And then it was like, murmurs amongst his friends—' James wiggles his fingers about, '—that he'd cottoned on about me and Bella. And then it turned into a scene from fucking *Platoon* because our lift home was just arriving and Whittaker was looking for me, and me and my friends jumped into the car and shouted *'Go go go!'* just as he came out the barn and sprinted at us. There was fucking dust flying.'

'At least you'll be away from here soon.'

He sips his glass of milk and nods. James, all being well with his A Levels, will be off to uni this autumn.

'I'm off to bed,' he says.

'Night night.'

I count the small number of complete days still separating me and the exams. They're on a Monday, Tuesday and Thursday. They're nearly here.

James's head reappears in the opening of the kitchen door. 'Did you hear about Dad?'

'Yeah,' I nod.

'Just checking,' and he dips back into the dark hallway.

'Has he said what he's going to do?' I ask.

James's face comes back into the light. 'Start a new company.'

32

It must be the food I eat that makes me nauseous every day. One of the books we're writing about in the Literature exam is *The Color Purple*, which has a moment where a character called Harpo, who gluts on pies to bulk up and match his wife in physical combat, leans over a rail and throws up what looks like a month's worth of food. Whenever I'm full or feeling sick I think about that image, and about all the things I've ate and drank mixing together, what it would look like back on the outside. I'm becoming afraid to eat much at all.

There are nights when Emma's round that I grow so nauseous I almost retch. She leaves not a moment too soon: I kiss her goodbye at the front door, holding it all down. She pulls herself away from me. I cover my mouth the second her back turns, trying not to hurl.[12]

I don't want you to think I'm just skiving, I type in an email to my personal tutor, and try to explain my absence as this lingering illness I can't shake.

33

Daylight, even when I wake up. The world's eyes are open.

Our bus pulls over on the journey to my first AS exam. More students get on, finding seats. I wipe my elbow across the

---

[12] 'Lurgee' by Radiohead revolves in my head: "I feel better. I feel better now you've gone."

condensation on the window and stare out at a pockmarked wall, stained with moisture from last night's drizzle.[13] The cool air, drawn through the open doors at the front of the bus, touches my face, and the doors close again.

From nowhere: a hot flush that reaches my fingers and toes, the sort you get moments before squeezing up vomit.

This is it. This is where it happens: halfway between college and home. I sit perfectly still and beg my body to have mercy. Not so much picturing the moment of projection as predicting it, planning where I'll aim, to make the least mess, be the least noticed.

A female voice asks if she can sit in the free seat beside me.

'Sure,' I mouth without looking up, and move my bag out her way and rest it on my feet. A pair of legs in caramel trousers sit down.

The bus lurches forward and every movement it makes slops my insides about. My stomach rises. I spent my desperate prayer in America.

But at this peak of sickness, the feeling ebbs away. Like a kettle clicking off when it hits boiling temperature, letting the water settle. A cautious relief, an empty weightlessness, spreads through me.

I dare to move. It's my chance to take some tablets. But this girl next to me will see. So, tipping a shoulder down to reach, my fingers trail blindly across the canvas of my bag, finding the cool of the side pocket's metal zip. Open it enough to fit the hand in and rifle through the tablet trays.

Not that one. Not that one.

Stemetil tablets are small and circular, on a hard, brittle tray, with a metallic foil.

Found it.

All the circular bubbles are depressed and emptied but one. It's been that way for months now, as taking the last Stemetil will leave none at all. And one day, I might need that last tablet even more

---

[13] Am I sick? I ask myself, check myself. Am I sick? Am I sick? Am I sick? Am I sick? Am I sick? Am I sick? I'm sure I can feel something. A stir. Am I sick? Am I sick? Am I sick? What about now? Am I sick? Am I sick?

desperately than today. So instead, let's find the painkillers. Larger, oblong shaped, in a malleable plastic tray with a more papery foil.

Here.

Pop two out – swallow them dry.

Is this a vicious cycle: always feeling sick *because* I take so many painkillers? They might help short-term but ultimately make things worse. "Drug fever", where your escalating symptoms are in fact the result of all the meds the doctors are throwing at your original complaint. They mentioned it on the *Scrubs* box set I played every night last summer to send myself to sleep. Will there be a quiet period – no college, no Emma – where I can stop taking painkillers?

Another surge of sickness. Blaring images flutter like insect wings: warm leftovers scraped into a bin bag; milk curdling and foam spreading inside me; yellow bile squirting up my throat; the reactions of passengers as my insides become my outsides; the sour pang of vomit wetting my taste buds; waiting, soiled, beside the road for a means home. It can't happen. My skin prickles.

I close my eyes. Try to think about clear trickling water, a bolted iron door, pitch darkness. Imagine the paracetamol soothing my insides, like in indigestion adverts, where the tablets turn into little firemen who put out the fires of stomach pain. It just thins the blood.

Even with my eyes shut, I know where we are by the turns the bus takes, and feel glimmers of comfort when we pass through an area of the journey with hiding places beside the road. I note each bump of the tarmac through the floor, through my seat, and mentally tick the checkpoints.

A loud *shump* sounds through the students' chatter.

I open my eyes.

Someone a few rows forward has stood and pulled their window open. The stream of air meets my face. People behind me complain but to me it feels incredible.

My body is made of objects I must consciously hold together, like I'm carrying an armful of potatoes. And I concentrate on not *spilling outwards* throughout each exam. Keep everything held together.

Keep the vomit down. After months of build-up, the worst never happens. Never mind what the test results will turn up; sitting there for three hours, three times without being ill was the goal.

As soon as it's "pens down" on the last exam it feels like a massive achievement to not drop all those spuds. Even if holding them forever is exhausting. I'm making no sense.

I pull my bag out the pile at the front of the hall, drop my pens in and head out into the sunshine, up the concrete steps and round the flower bed.

Is it really all behind me?

On the bus home, over the crop fields of the Ancholme Valley, I spot the cement works and the Humber Bridge beyond it. The fear falls away. What's left, when the thing I was scared of is over? Where does the worry go? That substance, that energy?

Ant meets me at the gym. We work out our chests and arms. He drinks protein and creatine all the time, takes a carton of boiled eggs to college every day, and his strength is inching ahead of mine.

'Do you hear that?' he shouts from the shower cubicle next to mine. 'I'm windmilling! You do it!'

'God, stop it,' I shout, noticing the wet slapping noise.

He announces that he's shaving all his hair off. I decide I want in, and that's our afternoon sorted.

In the concrete and corrugated plastic porch behind Ant's place, we take turns to shave each other's hair down to stubble with his mum's clippers.

For brief moments I feel free as a bird.

34

My friends plan a trip to the holiday house Boris's parents own in Sutton for a few nights in the summer holidays. I say I can't wait. And it's true: here, weeks away from the date, I want to go. I'll miss out if I don't go. But part of me already knows what will happen when it comes to it. When it stops being abstract, and becomes real, imminent. Every happy daydream of drinking on the beach, laughing all night, darkens into me being desperate to escape, being ill in front of my friends, who are drunk and laughing at me, *remembering*, as I stumble into the dark and run away, until the sun comes up and shows me, soiled and disgusting.

I'm already thinking of excuses to bow out.

35

For the first time I've known, Dad's no longer got a job. His old job is still there if he wants it, according to the new owner of Bright-Spec Windows. And to say Dad isn't *working* wouldn't be right either. Over the next week he scouts for a place to set up his new company, visits banks, answers calls from an endless list of clients and contractors he's worked with over the years. All the while, staff from Bright-Spec ring to see if they can come work with him if he manages to get set up.

It's also the first time I've known him without a company car. He goes out to buy a runabout and brings home an ancient, boxy Mercedes that we soon name The Hummer. I secretly feel sorry for him in that old thing; it's a big step down from the relatively modern Mondeo company car he had.

June brings its daily promise of hot weather. I spend a lot of time thinking about the long daylight hours and the heat of these next months.

'Happy birthday, fella!' Dad says when I come downstairs into the kitchen on a Monday morning. He pulls me into a hug and then goes 'Ha ha!' the way he does, patting my back.

Emma texts, asking me to go visit her for my present. I warn that I've only got an hour to spare because my grandparents are coming up for lunch.

Dad drives me there in The Hummer. 'I don't want to fall out with you,' he says, hitting my leg. 'Hey?'

'Me neither.'

Is he blaming me?

He talks on the phone for a mile or so. But it seems whoever's on the line can't guarantee Dad's new company any work.

'No, listen, that's fine,' Dad chuckles. 'No. Not a problem. Not a problem. You've got my number, anyway.'

'No luck?' I ask when he hangs up, thinking it better not to say he shouldn't use his phone whilst driving.

We enter Barrow, take a left at the roundabout where the face of Gordon Brown is stencil spray painted onto the traffic bollard.

'Not in this case,' he *ah-wells*.

'Will anyone who used to buy from you follow you over to the new company?'

'Oh yeah, some have already promised to. Many without me having to ask. I go a long way back with a lot of these guys. But some don't get to make those calls. It's going to be *bloody* hard.' On "*bloody*", he grips the wheel harder, juts his head forward with squinted eyelids, like the word itself is a barrier he smashes through. 'What're your plans this summer? We could really use an extra hand getting set up, if you're interested. You'll be paid, obviously.'

'Should be fine.' We pull into Emma's cul-de-sac and I look at the dashboard clock. 'Could you be here at twenty past twelve?'

'Yep. See you then. Alright,' he says as I'm getting out and saying bye.

Was he being nice because it's my birthday? The other week, Nanna had a quiet word with me about how me and Dad's fallouts are eating into him. Is it painful work to blank your son for months at a time?

I walk over the big square of grass to the end of the terrace, past the front yards of Emma's neighbours, who sit out on garden furniture and smoke, shouting over the low fences to each other. Emma's face appears in the kitchen window; she sees me open the picket gate, then dips behind the net curtains. I hear The Hummer pull away and picture touching down into a snake pit only to watch the rope ladder I climbed in on being raised out of reach.

'Happy birthday!' Emma yelps. She kisses me at the door then jumps back to let me in. Twirls her hips side to side with a big grin, in case I hadn't noticed she's wearing the brown skirt from when we first got together.

'Mm, nice.' I smile, closing the door and shuffling out of my trainers. 'You wearing that for me?'

'Yep.' She kisses me and takes my hand, leading me up the stairs.

My head swims from the sex; my face burns. We lie naked on top of the sheets. The window's ajar and a bit of air floats in and touches our damp skin. Our clothes are scattered about the floor.[14] It's quiet. I can hear the hamster gnawing the wooden toy in its cage, the neighbour's muffled dance music thudding through the wall, an engine ran-tanning far away in a farmer's field out the window. Emma's in my arms, which according to her letters is her favourite place to be. I pull her even closer and kiss the top of her head, catching the smell of her hair. Her little hand strokes over my ribs.

Downstairs, she hands me a card and says not to open it until later, and then presents, including a pack of Polos with a bow stuck to them. 'That one's a joke.' She giggles at my pretend stern look.

'This is all brilliant,' I say. 'Thanks so much.'

'Happy birthday,' she says again. 'Want a cuppa?'

'I think my dad's coming soon.'

'Ah. I'd better soak you up then.' She pushes her face into my chest.

---

[14] But my underwear doesn't directly touch the floor. Even in the heat of the moment I always tuck them inside my trousers. Floor bacteria. There's a system: my trousers can touch the floor, since sitting on the floor isn't unheard of. But I'd rather my t-shirt doesn't touch the floor, especially if there's somewhere I've got to be in the next day or so. My underwear mustn't touch the floor, but it also shouldn't touch my t-shirt, as my hands, which will then touch food etc., are likely to touch my t-shirt at some point, and if my underwear has rested on my t-shirt, it's like I've touched my junk before eating, right? My socks may touch the floor, and may touch the *outside* of my trousers, but not the inside of my trousers, because that would potentially transfer floor bacteria to my nether-regions, which may let it enter my body. My socks can't touch my t-shirt and they *certainly* can't touch my underwear. So I'll happily throw my clothes off in a suitably spontaneous and passionate way, but all whilst sticking to these rules.

Fifteen minutes later – but who's counting? – The Hummer arrives in the square outside. I say bye to Emma, who clings to my clothes on my way out. I kiss her again whilst twisting my ankles into my trainers.

In and out. I wish it was always like this. We got everything done: talking, laughing, kissing, sex, all a couple needs. Like watering a plant.

The skin lifts and flattens, lifts and flattens, catching the heat current and releasing it through a tear, a kind of breathing. Steam rises and my nose meets the smell. The fat leaks, hisses when it lands on the grey coals and leaves a dark splotch. Despite being scrubbed, the grill the chicken rests on is flecked with black remnants of meat from last year's barbecues. Little streaks of dark grease that even the scourer didn't catch. When I watch over it, my eyelids and forehead throb with the warmth.

We've got chairs out on the grass. Grandma, Granddad and Nanna sit in papery old people summer clothes, discussing the heat wave and the old families of Barton. Dad's given Nanna strict orders not to mention the Hobarts' underhand sale of Bright-Spec Windows. Jordan has the ability to sit and do nothing at all. His knees jiggle up and down – some of that restless energy kids have still lingers even at thirteen – but otherwise he only speaks when one of our grandparents ask him a question about school or his rugby team.

'Jordan!' Mum pokes when he isn't aware someone's speaking to him. Jordan snaps out of a daydream, his eyes doing that wide "I'm-paying-close-attention-and-I-swear-I-always-was" thing that cracks me up.

Dad's stood here at the barby with me.

Bentley the rabbit runs around our feet, rubbing his chin on our shoes and occasionally making love to the half-deflated football.

'What have we come for if not a booze-up?' Granddad jokes, taking the short glass of red Mum hands him. She returns inside, comes back out with a tray in each hand: cutlery, napkins, a bowl of Doritos and dips, nuts, a salad. She lays them on the plastic table.

Sits down, comments how precarious her chair feels on our sloped lawn.

'What we need is a patio,' Dad says to me. He presses the chicken with a metal spatula; the clear liquid squelches out and excites the coals below. 'Up to where we're stood, running all the way across the back of the house. It doesn't matter if we lose half the lawn, you lads have grown out of playing football back here anyway.'

'True,' I say.

'And somewhere down the line, once I get up and running, we'll have to see about a conservatory.'

'That'd be cool.'

Mum sips from a slender glass of Budweiser and rasps, 'Aaah.' She takes a clean butter knife and stirs the ice cubes round. She'd never been partial to lager until last year's trip to SeaWorld. She'll drink no more than a small bottle's worth, heavily diluted with ice.

The food's ready. I sit at my place and take a grilled chicken leg.

At Leggott you can buy a KFC knockoff called Dixie Chicken. Bethany once bit into crumbed chicken breast and it was pink inside. Yes, I can't stop thinking about college. About last winter, sneaking under the windows here. Hiding down the alley, crouched on the frozen mud. James saying, 'It just came over me out of nowhere!' after he was sick. I still think about it. I think about everything. The burning of my skin when my stomach threatens to empty itself. Harpo vomiting a month's worth of rich food over the porch banister. Me barely eating anymore. Nine Inch Nails. "God is dead and no one cares." Holding my palms under a hand dryer in the shitty Maggy May toilets because the noise is a tiny island of comfort. The E-Block disabled toilets, famous for a place to shag because no one goes there, making it a good place to hide. Breathing in the dust that plumes from a patted seat on the bus. The head-filling, sinister, endless blast of happy chatter. Emma saving a seat for me every time I get on. Her eyes following me as I approach. The doors folding shut with a hiss and a *shump*. Noting where the "Emergency: Open" button beside the doors are on each of the three models of bus we get. Wishing I was alone. Coming home early. My friends, who ask where I go, why I don't stay, and I don't have an answer. The college year's not finished yet, and there's another to go. It's eternal. I have to take a year off. It's a disaster. I need to... recover. I see myself: ill at college. Ill on the bus. Ill in front of my friends. Their eyes. Their fucking eyes, watching. Their memories, remembering me forever. Their words, spreading, spreading.

Something's **not right**.

Thank fuck we aren't off on holiday this summer. It's nearly a year since our second trip to Florida and I still have dream after dream that we're going back, and I wake up relieved as its fraudulent reality falls away. I think about all our holidays. Long car journeys to the South, the train into London, the two-hour bus ride between the airport and hotel in Majorca when I was five. What if I had to do that now?

I dip a stick of celery through some cream cheese and go inside.

'How about this?' I turn my laptop round to face Dad later in the evening, who's sat in his living room chair, covered in black binders.

'Good, yeah. I don't want the towers, though. Just the bridge, going like *this* over the words.' He gestures an arc.

'Cool.' I carry on. I'm helping design the logo for Dad's new company, Humber Window Solutions.

36

The exam period's over, and there are three weeks of the college year left. I barely attend one lesson. I get as far as the Maggy May a few times, before taking a bus to town or hurrying through the park in bright sunshine to catch the 350 to Barton.

One day, it's siling down when I leave home in the morning. I reach the end of the street and the rain already dribbles off my nose, runs behind my ears, creeps between my neck and the collar of my coat, finding the t-shirt beneath and making it stick to my shoulders. I could be warm and dry on the bus. But I take a right, away from the stop. Climb over the slimy fence into Top Field.

Walk fifty metres in, turn and watch the gap in the trees to see the double-decker go past. A small relief always comes over me at this point. But also shame. There's no way I can be on it now: it's gone.

My feet are wet. My coat is soaked and my t-shirt clings to my whole torso; my jeans darken over my thighs and calves. I walk the rest of the field, down the slope, into the trees. It must stop raining soon.

It doesn't.

Through Tree Field, past Death Hill and the old cauliflower field, the growing mound of mud, collected from the foundations dug beside it, is now sprouting grass and weeds. I climb the long slope towards the motorway bridge. My shoes are caked in mud and full of water. It's sucked through my toes and socks with every step. Tiny waterfalls trickle off the thick chods of turned soil, gathering to form a stream at the side of the field and pouring down to lower ground.

From the top of Barton I tramp down Horkstow Road, turn into the farmer's track. Chalk clumps peeking from the slimy mud are washed white. The thick tractor tyre gouges brim with water; I keep between them and try not to slip. Tread all the way to the bramble bank, off the track and up the next hill, well out of town now, then I cut into the low trees and weeds. The twig ends and thorns pull on my wet coat and more water splashes down when I disturb the branches.

This is the place I fingered Alicia when I was thirteen, and that makes me loathe being here, but I remember it being sheltered. A natural den, too low to stand straight but with a thick canopy of leaves above and around it. Back on that maddeningly exciting day, it was warm and dry, secluded, hardly classy, but I needed this place then in a vaguely comparable way to how I need it today: I can't be at home but I need shelter.

There's nowhere else, I think, taking my backpack off. My gym clothes are packed, and luckily in a plastic bag too, because a good pint of water has collected in the bottom of my backpack, ruining my books and pens. My collection of tablets in the side pocket – are the foil trays they are kept in waterproof? I pour the water out and put the clothes bag back in. I might as well have gone swimming: I can't get any wetter than this. I take my coat off and wring water out of it. Make to put it back on, but the wet material is so cold on my skin that I can't bear it. I set my bag down, and the coat on top of it, noticing that I'm shaking, my teeth chattering like the clappers. I can't sit because the ground is sodden mud, so I squat down, hugging myself. On the white skin of my arms it's hard to tell the droplets from the goosebumps.

Listen to the innumerable patters of rain hitting big green leaves. It's coming through the canopy. Not as much as being out in the open, but it's still coming through. I'd imagined being in here for a few hours and dripping dry – well *that's* gone tits-up.

A gust blows and all the leaves tip their collection down on me.

Bloated raindrops make crown-shaped splashes on the surface of a muddy pond that was once the gym's car park. I find a way round and head inside.

'Fucking hell,' Dean huffs behind the counter, his eyes widening.

'I know. This is just from between my house and here,' I lie. I've been nearly four hours in this downpour.

My shoes squelch through the gym and print a trail of dark splotches on the carpet. In the changing room I peel everything off down to my boxers and socks, wishing I'd thought to bring a change of them, too. Wring out my jeans, coat and t-shirt, open the sauna and hang them on the benches. Take out the bucket of water you'd spoon onto the coals and empty it in the kitchen sink. Hopefully that will keep the heat in there dry. The last thing I want to do is work out, but I can't stay here and do nothing.

The shaking doesn't stop and I'm weak as hell. The wetness from my boxers seeps through my jogging bottoms in a dark stain and leaves an arse print wherever I sit. 'Umbrella' by Rihanna plays on the wall-mounted TVs and I remember the upper level of the bus, the morning Sophia and her friends sung the "eh, eh, eh" part and laughed, their feet up on the rail, swiping mist from the front windscreen with the soles of their boots. How trapped I was. The song makes me aware of a gentle contraction of my throat, a nauseating, stodgy heat behind my eyes, just like on that day; like the tune of 'Umbrella' dredges up not only a memory of being there, but its very reality.

I catch my reflection and notice one hand's on my stomach, so I lower it. My gym top sticks to me, but I'm sure my arms aren't as thick as they were. Not like in the close-up picture I took last year and set as my phone background.

I open the sauna after nearly an hour and pat my clothes. They're no drier – just warm. That's the only difference. I take them out, lay them across the wooden bench surrounding the changing room, thinking of all the sweaty arse cracks that have been in contact with the places I'm laying my clothes. Take the paperwork, now melded into a single soggy cuboid, out my backpack and pour any residual water down the sink. The pocket ripped from a peg bag I made in Year Eight falls out. I wring it out and throw it back in.

Back in the gym, I manage a few more tricep exercises before thinking *fuck it.* Sit in the sauna for as long as I can, shower, realise I haven't brought a towel, stand in the cubicle and drip dry for a while. The trembling starts again. I wince to put the soaking clothes back on, but if I arrive home in gym gear and one of my parents are there, how would I explain it?

Green leaves, ripped prematurely from the trees, float on the car park's new pond. The water makes tight ripples when the wind skims its surface, as though it winces to the touch.

37

The whole country's flooding, according to the news Mum has on the following morning. She sits by the bay window, knees up to her chin, feet tucked under the chair's arm to her side. Every morning she puts a couple of tomatoes in boiling water to loosen their skin. Peels them, slices them, lays them on toast, adds salt and pepper. She stares at the TV now and chews this breakfast.

Water *pours* down the stairs of our bus. It bubbles up like a burst drain through the overlapping plates that make the flooring. Runs to the back when we accelerate, sloshes to the side when we turn. It trickles down the walls. Pisses through a gap in the ceiling onto a seat no one will go near. It's still raining outside but does that account for *this much* water?

We have to skip Winteringham. As we pass the turn-off we'd usually take to go there, you can see the whole road is submerged; a car is stranded and the brown water's up to its windscreen.

Me and Emma keep our bags off the floor. She sits hers on her lap but I think about how dirty the underneath of a bag is, and that dirt transferring to my jeans, so instead I hold it in front of me all the way there. It's dried out from yesterday and I've salvaged most of my work.

The floods are unusual enough to distract me and it's actually a pretty fun ride. But as we get closer to Scunthorpe, queasiness creeps in. I rehearse the smell and sound of the Maggy May. The image of that toast they sell behind the counter, soaked with butter, recurs in my head and I imagine the taste. That cheese toasty they do. Holding one above me and tilting my head to catch the drooling, milky cheese in my mouth. I imagine drinking loads and loads of milk. I imagine bread soaked in milk, disintegrating into an anaemic slop.

My scalp prickles.

At college, it's ten to nine and I set off from the Maggy May to first period Art, but once Emma breaks off to go to her Biology class I find myself ducking through the A-Block corridor, out the rear entrance and splashing towards town.

Patches of the park are flooded. Avoiding one pond only leads to another; paths disappear under water. I double back every time my foot sinks into waterlogged grass, increasingly desperate as ten past ten approaches.[15] I stare at a tree sticking out the floodwater and guess the depth. Surely it can't get any deeper than knee-high. I wade in.

---

[15] It *must* be this first bus. I have an hour to get home. It will all happen after an hour: vomiting, shitting, vomiting, shitting. If I miss this bus, I'll be abandoned in town centre for an hour. I can see the rushing ghosts watching me puke, making a wide berth of me there in the street. The silent disgust, the sympathy, the shuffling of feet to keep away from me.

38

Ant and me walk down to my grandparents' for an extra set of outdoor chairs and a table. As we cross the drive I raise a hand to Granddad, who's sat in the living room by the front window, as always. He doesn't wave back, but his head slowly turns, tracking us as we walk. His eyesight's terrible. We open the side passage gate, into the garden.

'Look. That's where I landed,' I tell Ant, pointing to a section of hedge beside us that's splayed and broken. 'I dived into it off the wall when we lived here in Year Seven.'

'Ooh, you rebel. You jackass.' Ant shakes me.

Grandma's got the plastic furniture out on the grass by a bowl of suds, wiping them with an old white dishcloth. You know, the netted sort no one uses anymore.

She dabs her forehead with a wrist, shakes her head at us with a stern look, then laughs.

'We could've cleaned them!' I say.

'Well, *go on then*,' she says, thrusting me the rag. 'I'd better check on The Boss.' She potters inside.

We scrub green scum off the chairs, accumulated from the permanently damp shade behind the house, then tip them up to dry.

It's all for a party I'm hosting, an hour from now.

Emma wishes it was her, rather than Ant, seeing me before everyone arrives. But I was nervous, shut in my room playing *Ghost Recon*, nauseous and wondering whether to cancel the whole thing.[16] Then Ant arrived, and he's so… *simple* that it comforts me. Not "simple" as in stupid: I just mean he's happy and calm. He doesn't need things. Doesn't need to cuddle, kiss and hang off me like Emma does.

---

[16] Repeatedly picturing being sick and having to run inside whilst all my friends watch, ask questions, come to find me, even laugh. But why do I care, when a party is a rare instance where it's alright to be sick?

I nip inside my grandparents' house, through the utility room that always smells of detergent powder and the freshly snapped stem of a plant. Grandma stands at the kitchen sink. She flicks water from her veiny fingers into the basin, then dries them on a tea towel. Drapes the towel over the side of the sink, and a quarter of it rests in the soapy water. She shuts the microwave door. Leans on the counter and places a hand on her hip. 'And how's Christopher?'

'Good.'

'You'd better go see what The Boss has to say. I'll make sure your friend isn't causing trouble.'

Their hallway carpet's yellow and trodden flat. The grandfather clock *chick-chock*s the seconds away, only the intervals feel like more than a second.

Granddad turns away from the lounge window and laces his fingers together. 'And what brings you here?'

'Not much. I've just come to get the chairs. We're gonna carry them up the hill back to mine.'

'Ah!'

'We'll take good care of them.' I smile.

He smiles, too. 'I should hope so. So what's been happening with you, hmm?'

'Oh, not a lot, really.'

His enthusiasm makes me feel bad for having to leave straight away, but I can't leave Ant in the garden. Since I've grown older, Granddad happily keeps me here for hours, talking about ancient history. He will first ask how my education is going. Then he will introduce a local subject like the building of Lincoln Cathedral and Thornton Abbey, the life of Havelok the Dane, old Lincolnshire vernacular, patterns of bell ringing, or further-reaching topics like the translational errors in the English Bible, comparisons showing how the current wars in the Middle East mirror those that have been happening for hundreds – or thousands – of years, the building methods of other famous monuments. He gives an introduction and then asks, 'Does that interest you?' Almost like he's a book I read the blurb of before deciding whether to open it. It's not like I'm going to say no.

Important friends from mysterious fraternities come over to discuss academic shit deep into the afternoons, consulting Granddad's library of books and journals. Granddad left school at fourteen and educated himself for seventy years. But he must lose track of who he's said what to, because he's repeated certain subjects to me dozens of times. I'll sit and say, 'Oh right!' again nonetheless.

Today, I only perch on the arm of the sofa, knowing that if I sit down properly, I'll be kept here no matter who's waiting for me in the garden.

'Very good. Don't forget our address,' Granddad says when I make my excuses and stand up.

I close the back door behind me and show the whites of my eyes to Ant, who grins. He takes the stack of six chairs; I carry the table. We say bye to Grandma and set off.

'Your granddad thought I was your girlfriend,' Ant says.

'What?'

'Your nan told me.'

'Oh right,' I say. 'His eyesight *is* pretty bad. But I don't know who that's more insulting for. Are you womanly, or is Emma butch?'

He laughs. 'I'm like twice Emma's height. If his eyesight's blurry, I bet you and Emma look like fucking Lennie and George coming down the drive.'

'They've never met her.'

A dozen friends arrive. I stoke up the barbeque, wheel out a set of speakers and put an iPod playlist on. Fill a bucket with cold water for the beers. The two tables are put together and we sit around them eating and drinking. We alternate who stands by the hot coals, turning the meat. Boris puts his bare, mud-stained feet up, Ben has a scarf drooped round his tiny shoulders despite it being summer, James plays guitar. I stand behind Emma and put my hands on her shoulders. She puts her palm over one and keeps talking to Bethany. Jordan quietly eats with us beside his even quieter friend I said he could bring along. Sebastian hides behind his SLR camera, taking arty shots of the party. I poke a leaf of salad through the wire mesh of the rabbit hutch and Bentley pulls it from my fingers. We get out a yard-of-ale glass, funnel-shaped with a spherical bottom. Ant tries to drink a full yard whilst I film with my digital camera; it takes him so long that someone comments, 'It looks like you're playing a trumpet.' He chokes and beer gushes out his nose. Boris refills it and necks it down, no problem. I sit at the table later and watch the film back. Right near the microphone, you can hear Ben singing along to 'Go to Sleep' by Radiohead that plays in the background.

Emma leans her head on me and I turn the camera screen for her to see. I wonder why on earth I almost cancelled this party.

Jordan and his mate disappear when the drinking games start.

Dale drinks a forfeit of King Jug shitmix, and his attempt is so terrible that Sebastian mumbles, 'Dale, you drink like old people fuck.'

'Eeyore's a bitch when he's had his two beers,' Ant laughs.

The late afternoon turns to evening and we move inside. Emma makes a show of being comfortable, wandering through to other rooms, talking to my parents more confidently than usual, offering people drinks or showing them where to find certain things. Marking her territory.

When everyone's packed around the kitchen table, she gets up and squeezes between the tangle of chairs. Her eyes wait for mine to meet them as she pulls the kitchen door to behind her, but I don't look across.

Sebastian strums on James's guitar, head hanging as Cobain-esque as he can over the strings. Ant and Ben begin a rally of "your mum" jokes that lasts nearly half an hour, until my abdomen aches from laughing.

I go upstairs and open my bedroom door. There's just enough twilight left outside to illuminate the blinds a grey colour. Emma's in my bed. I kneel beside it and stroke her hair. 'Hey. You okay?'

'Yeah,' she says. 'Sounds like you're having fun down there.'

'Are you coming down?'

'I was waiting to see you first.'

'Oh aye?' I kiss her jawline and shoulder.

'Not like that,' she says.

But I put my hand under the covers, stroke her jeans for a couple of seconds, move into her underwear, shrugging my shoulder up to make the awkward angle, and discover that, well, she wasn't lying. I retract my hand.

'Are you okay?' I say again.

'Sure,' she says, and tells me something about coming up here because her head hurt, and wanting five minutes of me to herself, but I'm busy feeling embarrassed that I failed to immediately turn her on, and ashamed I hadn't taken her seriously enough when she'd said 'Not like that'. I hadn't even wanted to take it further; I imagined we'd playfully tease each other for a minute before we went downstairs together. How arrogant am I, to think she'd just melt and no longer feel down about whatever's bothering her if I stick my hand down her pants? It's hopefully too dark to see me blush.

'I can stay with you a while,' I say.

'Everyone's here, though.'

'I don't mind.'

'No, come on.' She gets up. I stand and she hugs me. 'Thanks for being nice,' she says, though I don't feel like I was nice at all.

We emerge back into the group, blinking in the light, greeted with a loud, accusatory '*Waheeey*!' that makes Emma laugh and say, 'I was just tired!'

Later on we put wood on the smouldering coals of the barbeque and get a fire going. James sits on the grass and plays guitar, and Bethany watches him with doughy eyes. Once most people leave, me, Emma and Boris hang out in my room. Emma and Boris both live in Barrow, and I've persuaded Emma to let Boris hitch a ride home with her mum. This way, I don't have to spend any time with her alone, and she can't mention sleeping over.

I turn on the Xbox and play the stored music whilst we chat. The visualiser on the screen swirls and pulses glass shapes, zooms up and down psychedelic tunnels, phasing through kaleidoscopic patterns of every colour. Five and a half minutes into 'Us and Them' by Pink Floyd, as the saxophone jams away, Boris tilts his drunk head back and goes, 'That is *gorgeous*.'

39

The problem with sleepovers was never the dark. It was the point of no return that you pass, almost literally.

A primary school friend once stopped over and then had a mild asthma attack at midnight, which, at eight years old, felt like the very dead of night. We had to wake my parents, who called his dad, who then seemed to take an age to get over from the next village with the inhaler.

When Ryan and Ben were round on the night before my eleventh birthday – the night I saw a ghost, incidentally – I felt terribly sick but knew I couldn't ask them to leave at that time; it would've taken phone calls to parents, waking people up.

I slept at friends' houses and felt the break-off point, when it was suddenly too late to go home. As though the world goes to sleep at night, and to stay awake into that time is to trespass, that wherever you are you must stay until morning, lest you wake the adults.

Even growing up, when sleeping out got easier, I would still feel like we'd lost our mooring and drifted away from shore once it passed half eleven. In the numerous "tenters" Ben hosted, I would repeatedly tell myself, *Look, if you wanted to, you could walk home any time*, but also not believe it. I didn't have a house key and would land in trouble to turn up at my house and knock sheepishly on the door at two in the morning. My way of getting through this was to stay awake all night. When the sun rose, I knew my parents would be awake and ready to receive a phone call, should I want to leave.

I remember waiting for that time desperately one night over at Morgan's, after playing with the gerbils, fending gypsies away from his front door, watching *The Matrix Reloaded* and *The Exorcist* on pirate DVDs in sleeping bags in front of the TV with Alicia sharing mine. I spent the early hours with a painful stomach, which led to taking a massive shit in his toilet, semi-visible to Alicia through the obscured glass door. I just wanted the glacial hour hand to hurry past six so that my parents would be awake to come rescue me. And as soon as I left, I felt fine.

Bitty would never sleep out, and everyone used to make fun of him. Secretly, I wished I could ask him why, and tell him I didn't like it either. Shortly after, I stopped staying out. Always making excuses, usually throwing my parents under the bus. Pretending I was grounded. And without me, the tenters seemed to fizzle out and stop happening.

As alcohol started trickling its way into our weekends, it made me all the more grateful to escape when it got late, trudge home and do some writing on the family computer or listen to my iPod on my bed whilst my head was fuzzy. Feeling completely alone and completely safe.

A couple of years ago, after a gig at The Carnival, me and Ben stayed out in his summerhouse, at the top of his long garden, and then I decided to go home at three in the morning. I walked back in the dark and drizzle. At this point I kept a stolen key to our patio door, and knowing Mum was in the next room asleep on the sofa, I spent no less than twenty minutes turning the key, opening the door, parting the blinds, stepping in, removing my shoes and sneaking up to my room. I lay in bed wondering how in the morning I could explain why I was here.

In the last year of school, a girl who kept horses and had loads of land threw a monstrous party in Barrow Haven, thirteen minutes from home. Tents were pitched everywhere. It was late spring and it seemed to stay light for ages. I hooked up with a girl from a different school. She knew I wasn't staying the night, and spent the whole evening trying to convince me otherwise. 'Stay,' she said, simply. Almost a beg. 'Stay.' Between kisses, after zipping her tent up behind us. Letting my hands find her breasts. 'Stay.' Big eyes, surrounded with black liner. I knew what staying would lead to, but even that didn't drown out the thought of being stranded out here, so at midnight, as arranged, Dad picked me up. Ryan told me the following Monday that he'd then gone into that tent for, as he worded it, "sloppy seconds".

Emma's text reads: *I love it when you can hear the rain at night. it's so relaxing xxxxx*. I close my flip phone, feel for my bedside table and set it down. I was just lying here enjoying the sound of rain on the windowsill myself. She knows I love the sound of rain. Is she copying me for affection? So I think we have more in common? She is that sort of person. No, I think she's really thinking about rain. And I find myself longing to be next to her, enjoying it together. It hurts that I can't bring myself to sleep with her. Time's ticking by. I don't let anyone else know, and I worry what Emma says to others. It's a central part of any relationship and I haven't done it yet. Emma wants to, so much, but never makes a meal of it. I turn over. That text makes me think how harmless she is.

College has finished for the year.

I've no idea if I'm going back.

Having a year out is an idea Mum doesn't like the sound of. 'I think if you get a job or work with Dad you'll get used to getting a little income, and never go back to college at all,' she says one morning, stood against the counter eating tomatoes on toast, holding the little plate right up beneath her chin to catch any crumbs. 'You have to remember though, your income won't ever increase much unless you at least finish your second year of college and get some qualifications under your belt. This job you get might be *it* for you, and that's a long, long flat road, all the way to retirement.'

'People do the whole "gap year" thing all the time.'

'While they're at uni, maybe. I don't know about many taking a year off halfway through college.'

'I'd definitely go back. I just need time off.'

'You've got six or seven weeks off ahead of you,' Mum says, but I'm not sure she gets what I mean.

I don't fully get it either.

Whatever it is going wrong with me, I remember being this way when I was little, like eight or ten years old. Then, it was a fear of needing to use the toilet whilst being out somewhere. It went away because I got older, but equally because – compared to the military strictness of primary school – Baysgarth didn't pose much to fear. Only the very rare school trip, which yes I dreaded, even if I couldn't pinpoint why. But for the most part, that big break from things to worry about let me heal; and now that I'm at college it's come back, because I'm always so far from home. That's my reason for wanting this next year off. I've got a feeling that whatever's happening to me will go away, given time to rest from worry. It seems a sensible solution.

Emma will still want to see me though.

My parents will still want me to go places with them.

Mum continues her speech about me completing my education. It goes on until her toast's finished, her plate and chopping board are washed and set out to drip dry, the toaster put away. I'm sat on the chair, sometimes listening, sometimes dreaming.

From the hall Dad shouts, 'You fit, Chris?'

'In here,' I call.

He comes in, re-tucking his shirt into his jeans and smiling. I pour the dregs of my tea down the sink and follow him outside to The Hummer. It's a cool and clear morning. Barton's gotten off lucky after the floods. Only the areas closest to the Humber flood-plains have their doors sandbagged and their downstairs ruined.

We trundle through town to the workshop Dad's renting at the east edge of Barton. The clock strikes eight: Humber Window Solutions is officially open.

'What I'm thinking… is a compressor *here*.' Dad gestures with both hands to the corner of the empty workshop. His voice is loud and reverberates off the high corrugated walls. 'Work benches: *shum, shum*.' He makes chopping gestures where things will go. 'Room for three pairs of trestles. V-notch, corner welder, T-welder, copy router: *shum, shum*. Cagger can go on the bench.' He scratches his head with one finger, rotates on his heel and grimaces in thought. I've no idea what he's talking about. 'Come on,' he says. He walks about faster than I know him to, and for some reason whistles the jingle of a comedy channel we watch in the mornings and the chorus of Robbie Williams's 'Rudebox' through his front teeth.

By the entrance is a little office. Granddad's old desk, plan trolley and drawing board have been moved in. A phone waits on the hook. A stack of black folders lean against the wall. Dad sits behind the desk and smiles.

'What do you think?'

The next few days see the machinery being delivered. 'It's pre-owned stuff,' Dad points out. 'Older than you are, I'd bet. But it's more than capable.' Plastic arrives in six-metre extruded lengths that we store on metal racks. We calibrate the machinery. Each link in the chain of production has to work in a very exact way. One must add *this* much, the next must shave off *this* much, burn off *this* much, be set at *this* angle, apply *this* much pressure. And every time the compressor senses the machines need more air pressure, it blasts into life like a decrepit Harley and I jump out my skin.

Dad shows me how to make a basic window, but only in ten-minute bursts before he runs into the office to answer the phone again, and doesn't come back out for the next hour, tending to whatever the call was about. I'm left without a clue and sweep the floor. Brush lint off the green metal of a welder. Smell rust on my fingertips. Sharpen a pencil with a Stanley knife. I do my best not to snap at Dad's patronising teaching. One frame and sash takes two days to make. I have to man the office phone whenever he goes out. Callers mistake my voice for his and start yapping about windows before I get chance to correct them and take a message. On the notepad beside Dad's ancient calculator I write a couple of new paragraphs for the post-apocalyptic story I began a few years ago. Everyone dies at the end and the bad guys win. Man, Nine Inch Nails is like the *soundtrack* to it. I picture it being made into a film, *The Fragile*'s 'Underneath It All' sounding in the end credits.

We nip to the printers for a stack of letterheads and business cards. Dad sets up a company account with the printers whilst I play with the different pens. 'The sign for the workshop should be coming next week,' he tells me, opening the door that still knocks a bell on the jamb. 'A guy in Scunny hand-paints them.'

A week later, my school form tutor and P.E. teacher Patrick Scatcliffe visits in his blue, chip fat-fuelled truck. He's my dad's best friend and used to frequently join him in not speaking to me. Patrick puts the work benches together, makes a noise shelter for the compressor and requests the first order for Humber Windows: a small side-opening window for his back bedroom. I spend the day trying to make it, cocking up time after time. When I get pissed off with a mistake that sets me back six hours, he and Dad make jokes about teenage hormones and laugh to each other.

40

I count down the days to Emma going on a two-week holiday with her family.

Our friends come round to hang in the garden for her last night. And after they leave, Emma and me head up to my room, have sex on the floor, then lie on top of the covers of my bed with the window wide open. One of those nights where the moon is bright and every star is out. I kneel up on the bed, lean my shoulders out the window and study how the moonlight even casts a shadow of the fence and washing pole. 'Isn't it weird,' I say.

Emma manoeuvres under the covers and pretends to sleep. I tuck in behind her. Being so much shorter than me, when we spoon like this she fits perfectly into my torso. 'My favourite place,' she says. 'Are you going to miss me?'

'Nope.'

She tuts.

'Of course I'll miss you,' I say, quite sure it's a lie. 'It's only a fortnight, though.'

I can't wait for the moment she's out the door. I've been picturing all the things I can do without her. Go see my friends without having to organise how she'll fit into my plans. Leave places whenever I want to. Send texts to her without risking her suggesting we meet up. It's like a dozen deadlines getting postponed.

'It makes me think about this time next year. I've thought about it a lot, lately,' she says. 'We'll probably be off to uni that September, and it isn't likely we'll end up at the same one.'

'Yeah?'

'We should think about what we're going to do. This girl from Psychology has a deal with her boyfriend that they'll break up before they go to uni because it's less painful than it slowly coming to bits while they're apart. I didn't know if you think about that at all.'

'I haven't, really.' A tiny drop of adrenaline lands in my blood. 'What do you think?'

Her voice goes up a note. 'I don't want to break up.'

'Me neither, so that's settled. I bet we'll be fine.'

She sighs and squeezes my arm. 'Good.'

What's this? Relief? For a moment there I thought she was suggesting we made the same arrangement as her friend. I shouldn't care either way if she wanted to break up with me. I'm a lone wolf. Don't *ever* wind up in a position where you need to be with somebody.

41

In the days, I work at Humber Windows, trying to learn the simplest tasks in window-making. Constantly frustrated and *so* fucking bored. But at least I'm saving some money. Five pound an hour, nine hours a day, and the days soon add up.

In the evenings I play Xbox with Jordan or go down to Ben's. A small group of us will sit on the patio beside his pond, and the sun will still shine down the lawn at half eight.

Marshall dangles two zip-lock bags of drugs up and down like yo-yos. 'Both legal. Fully endorsed. Got 'em online.' When he grins I'm reminded how brown his teeth have turned in the short year he's been on the herbs. 'Alternative to weed,' he says, holding up one bag. 'Hallucinogen,' he says, holding up the other, before barking into laughter that turns into a cough. He spits on the floor, and it looks like someone's stirred their finger through a splat of raw egg.

Ben holds a penny with barbeque pincers; everyone else holds lighters beneath it until the penny emits a faint glow. Ethan lets us hold his arm down on the glass table. Ben asks 'Are you *sure*?' then drops the penny onto the back of Ethan's hand. Everyone shouts in joy and horror, jumping to our feet, holding our heads. Ethan keeps quiet and doesn't move, his mouth open, sucking in air between grinding teeth. Smoke comes off his hand. His chair scrapes and he jumps up, shaking his wrist. The penny's stuck on. 'The fucking skin!' I shout. The penny hangs off by a flap and then drops out of sight.

'Agh, Jesus,' Ethan says with all the urgency of someone who's just squeezed the watery first helping of ketchup all over their chips. He lays his arm on the table and everyone leans in to inspect the raw, glistening, perfect circle left on his hand. 'You've no idea how much this hurts,' he says.

I'm so happy Emma's not here.

* * *

'Just because we're seventeen now, it's not like we can't still do this kind of shit,' Morgan says, his thick fingers smearing combat paint across his cheeks in the near-dark.

'Absolutely,' I say.

Ten of us are dressed in our darkest clothes in Top Field, by the edge of the trees. Marshall's brought some camouflage paint he got in the Territorial Army: brown, green and black in little shoe polish tins. We laugh at Wykes, who completely blacks-up his face, except his pale eyelids and lips. I'm in dark jeans, a thin black jumper and wool hat. I draw the paint under my eyes and we head down into the trees.

The game is "Trackers". First, we pick a "base" tree. In this case, the burned tree where we used to do turbos, where Ryan once got stuck hanging off a branch because his sovereign ring got caught under a flattened nail. This is where five people have to reach, without the other five spotting them. If a tracker sees you, they shout your name and you're out.

It's nearly ten o'clock and the sun's down. Away from any street-lights, it's got *really* dark. I'm on the sneaking team.

'Want to stick together?' says Bitty.

'Na, I'm okay.' I jog further into the trees and leave him behind.

Tree Field is a network of grass pathways lacing through dense areas of young trees. Where the mowers can't reach, weeds and bushes grow and the grass is waist-high. Were it daytime, you could look through the trees and see that cobwebs span between every trunk, see the hundreds of fat-bottomed spiders waiting.

But spiders concern me less than the tramps who occupy scorched clearings deeper within the trees. And the tramps concern me less than the supernatural. Even at seventeen, I jump when I think I see something in the dark, when the wind forms a momentary figure out of a bush, like a standing or crouching man, when it hisses through the trees and I hear a voice.

I go off the path and wade a few yards into the weeds, crouch down on one knee, pull a cobweb from under my chin. Another flurry of wind rolls through the bushes. The spindly treetops whip about and then settle. It's darker and quieter than I'm used to; it's brilliant. Hiding makes me need a piss but I keep still.

What if everyone's gone? It's been quiet for a long time now. I listen for the cars, a couple of hundred metres away, over the bank, that *swish* by on the dual carriageway. It would be a reminder that humans are still here. But the wind masks them. I swap knees. A few of my mates were pretty nervous about splitting up into the dark; maybe everyone went back and forgot about me.

My eyes can make out the path I'm overlooking. Thick, flattened clumps of grass coated in a wet film, like slicked comb overs.

Marshall's shout floats over the trees. 'Got you, Morgan.'

After another spell of quiet I notice faint thuds of footsteps coming my way. I crouch lower. Wykes and Webster trudge past, only a step from where I hide. I wait for them to spot me but they keep walking. They whisper, slightly out of breath. Their footsteps fade away.

Now's my chance to make a break for the burned tree. But for a few more seconds, I enjoy being invisible here in the undergrowth.

42

On the second week Emma's away she tells me she's counting down the days to seeing me again.

Me too, I reply.

I make a larger window for Baysgarth School; it takes nearly three days, and then Dad has to finish it anyway.

'Harvey's fitting it tomorrow. Do you fancy mucking in with him?'

'Sure,' I say, and that's all I think about for the rest of the day.

Baysgarth is one road away from work. A two-minute trip. And obviously walking distance from home. But the moment I get into Harvey's van the next morning I feel a hot wash of sickness come over me. My mouth purses and chews. I mentally rehearse excuses to jump out, but I'm stuck. We set off and I close my eyes.

We park the van in the bus circle and walk through the empty school. Harvey carries the window frame; I bring the tools. Over the concrete tennis courts, I see the yellow railings of The Corner, where me and my friends hung out for five years. In the forever-damp courtyard below the Maths block that stinks of drains, Harvey spots a used condom amongst the litter on the ground. 'Naughty boy!' he says, poking it with the tip of his boot.

He spends the morning scraping putty off the existing window to get the glass out. And the afternoon cutting some metal rod that's in his way. With his head tilted back, squinting at the ceiling, you can see right up his nostrils. I sweep the floor and avoid the grinder sparks. At four, he announces that we're done for the day. It's the least I've ever done whilst working at Dad's. Normally my feet ache by now. Part of me feels cheated.

That evening at Ben's, things get weird. What begins as a couple of challenges – who can take the most punches to the shoulder, for example – turns into Boris drinking paint water from Ben's Warhammer table, Morgan getting his arse smacked raw with the heel of a Converse sneaker, me getting a cigar put out on my forearm. At one point, Ant holds Wykes's arms back whilst Ryan slaps his bare stomach until a red hand mark starts to appear and Wykes laughs in pain. Ryan then pauses mid-strike, his arm raised, as though suddenly seeing the full picture. He turns to us and says, 'This is getting really gay.'

On Saturday we put our very best clothes on, light a barby in Morgan's garden and get drunk all afternoon.

Ant finds me stood over the barbeque, turning burgers that are so cheap half of them disintegrate between the grill.

'I can't believe you can't come tomorrow,' he says.

'It's shit.' I take a pull of my cigarillo, a bite of my burger, a sip of my beer.

Everyone's going to Sutton. I've fed them some excuse about having to help my dad get set up or having to do college work – I can't even remember. They keep going through the plan: Boris's mum picking up four people; Ben's dad picking up the other five in his people carrier; Webster, the only one of us with half a car, following behind two hours later with everyone's booze. It's an hour and thirty-minute drive.

When I was seven, a friend's mum took a bunch of us bowling in a big people carrier for her spoilt son's birthday party. 'Excuse my armpits,' she said, leaning over us, jiggling each of our seatbelts in their clips, in case we hadn't fastened them right ourselves, I supposed. The journey felt endless. The close laughter so loud. And even then, my own shouting and laughing, the whole bottle rocket scene, became muffled behind a translucent screen; I was on the other side, thinking about the toilet, whether I needed to go, and a panic was swelling. Laughing on the outside and fucking sobbing on the inside.

* * *

Emma arrives home. She sits me down at her dad's computer under their stairs, sits on my knees and starts the slideshow of photos from their holiday down south. My eyes track to the clock at the bottom right corner of the screen. A minute passes and I'm one minute closer to being picked up at five. How does the Shakespeare quote go? "Time passes, come what may", or something along those lines. It was painted on the wall of an English classroom back in school, and I think about it still. It's encouraging to know time keeps moving, no matter what. But other quotes make me uncomfortable. There's a moment in *Star Wars: Attack of the Clones* where C3PO is being thrown about through a factory and he exclaims, 'It's a nightmare!' and I hear those words when I'm in a terrible situation.

A photo of Emma sat on top of a gigantic black cannon at some castle they visited. In the right of the photo is her dad and big sister. Her sister's laughing at something her dad's saying. Her dad's face is in a smudged blur of movement. I imagine what it would've been like if I was there – because I *was* invited – trying to sleep in the campsite, Emma's family able to hear my every move through the thin caravan walls. Emma wanting to cuddle me. My heart beating. Holding in vomit and shit whilst the thought of how many uncrossable miles lie between there and home blasts in my ears like a trumpet in the dark. Emma's dad announcing that we're off on an hour's drive to see a castle in the morning.

It's a nightmare!

'Christopher,' Mum calls from the living room. 'Quick.'

I run into the lounge where she's got the local news on, holding the remote in her hand.

'Isn't this the mother of the two girls you and James know?' she asks.

The camera follows a woman being rushed beside a building towards its entrance, holding a bag or portfolio to shield her face from the cameras. The headline points out the irony: a counsellor for DUI offenders caught drink-driving. Loses job, faces charges. It's Sophia's mum. She used to tell me her mum was a drinker. The frightening ways it changed her. At Bradshaw's party, after school finished forever, whilst Nelly Furtado's 'Man Eater' squelched out of a broken speaker, I took Sophia aside and finally told her I wanted us to be together, and she began to cry. She told me her life was too fucked up; she didn't want me drawn into her problems. She hugged me. 'I already know about your problems,' I said over her shoulder. 'You've told me. I want to help. I want to be with you anyway.'

'But I don't want that for you,' she said.

'Is that her, then?' Mum asks now.

I write an email, hesitating, deleting and rewriting every sentence as I go. *You don't have to reply, and this isn't my place anymore, but I've seen the news and I'm so sorry*, it goes. I offer to help if there's any way I can.

I don't expect a reply – Sophia stopped replying to me back when she had the ear operation and became popular, and she'll be out doing something cool, not checking a computer for emails – but it arrives before night.

Your email made me cry. In a happy way, I think, she writes. It's thrilling to hear from her, a whole year after I ended our friendship. To know she has taken the time to write this. She explains what happened, and the aftermath in her house. I don't reply, despite the ache to. There's no way she will reply a second time. I'd rather take the ball and go home whilst it's in my court.

For the second attempt, I cut the sash profile, double-check the measurements, take the lengths back to my bench. Measure into the middle of the surface where the handle will be. Set up the router to drill the right holes.

Dad comes out the office.

'I've got to nip to Winterton to measure a job up. Want to come with?'

'Yeah.' I blast the plastic swath off me with the blower and follow him out.

We pass the sign that says "Winterton: 8 miles" as we leave Barton. Eight miles of A-road, which a car can do in fifteen minutes.

'It's at the fire station there. We're meeting the project supervisor. He's with North Lincs council. I've worked with him for many a year and luckily he wanted to keep in touch. This could be really good, keeping on his radar,' Dad says.

I'm okay when a small trip like this is sprung on me. It's like there isn't time to worry about it: you just go.

Emma wants to see me tonight.

Like with working out, if I let two days pass without seeing Emma, I start to feel the pressure; if I let three days pass, I get antsy, as though we'll drift apart. After seeing her, I feel a massive wave of relief, thinking, *that'll keep her going for a couple of days*; after a day or two have passed, I think, *I should probably see her again*; when, like today, she asks to see me only the day after our last meet-up, I think, *Jesus, again? I only saw you last night. Haven't I done my duty?*

Dad parks up outside the fire station. He reaches behind us and takes a notepad, pen and calculator from the back seat. Puts his reflector coat on and leads me round the side of the building, whistling 'Rudebox'. Shakes hands with who I guess is the supervisor and introduces me as "son number two" which always makes me happy.

On the drive home, Dad talks about upcoming work, things that need doing. How involved does he want me to be?

'Your mother told me you've been thinking about skipping college this year.'

'Thinking about it.'

A deep breath. 'If you wanted to work for me, the answer's yes. There is work for you. But it wouldn't be "come and go as you please". You'd be employed properly, on the books. Eight 'til five, Monday to Friday.'

'Would you want that?'

'It's not a question of what I want, Chris.' But then he answers, 'No. I want you to finish college at least. *At least* finish college. You've come this far, you've done well at school. I mean, is this all you want? To work here? And I know you say you'll go back to college in a year, but will you? The amount of times I told myself I wanted to go back into education, but once you're out Chris it's bloody hard to get back into it. You've got so many opportunities. I know that's what everyone says, but you do.'

No, I don't want to work for Dad for a year. Every day is like a fucking eternity in that workshop. But what's the alternative, really?

No one would want to hire me when I'm perpetually ill; it doesn't seem like I have many opportunities at all.

'Mum's off work next week. We were thinking of taking a ride out to Spurn Point one day before James leaves. What do you reckon?'

'Sounds good,' I say, whilst thinking, *shit*.

43

My latest bedroom arrangement's a pretty good one. The old computer table running across one wall, with the Xbox, monitor and speakers set up on it, and a gap for my laptop. It looks tidy, but I worry it makes me seem like a nerd. Who ever sees this room but Emma, though?

The Saturday arrives when we're off to Spurn Point, a long, thin peninsula, east of Hull, at the mouth of the Humber, apparently. All morning, I've stayed here in my room, hoping they for some reason forget I'm here. I bottled out of an Art class trip to Spurn Point last Easter, but I think I can manage this one. I play on Photoshop for a while. Hear Mum downstairs say, 'Just waiting for the washing to spin, and then we'll get going.'

My stomach flips. Oh God. No, I can't do it.

My door opens. 'Are you somewhere near?' Dad says.

'Yeah,' I say.

I go clean my teeth. Maybe the mint taste will make me feel better. Change my top, as though I intend to go. But at some point I'll have to tell them I can't. I'm scared shitless of that moment, whether it'll go down alright or spark another row like the night of the uni presentation. But I'm more scared of Spurn Point. Over the bridge, past Hull, further, further. I stand in the middle of my room, rubbing my temples with the base of my thumbs. Picture desperately needing the toilet out there, with no toilet in sight; picture needing to be sick, but we can't pull over.

'Ready?' Dad says. Behind him, I hear James and Jordan heading downstairs.

'Yeah,' I say, but don't move.

He sighs. 'What?'

I stay frozen. 'I don't think I can go.'

That stare I can't meet. Then, 'Chris, come on. Now. Move.'

'I don't think I can.'

He starts to turn round but then comes back in, like he's reset the conversation. 'Come on, let's go. Everyone's ready. *Chris*!'

'I *can't*.'

'Why?'

'I don't feel good.'

He goes away and I sit on the edge of my bed. Cover my mouth with my fingertips. I hear Dad telling Mum. I hear James say, 'What's going on?' downstairs at the front door. Footsteps coming up the stairs. I brace myself.

It's Mum. 'What's happening?'

'I can't go.'

'Why?'

'I don't *know*.'

'It's a half-hour drive,' says Dad, appearing behind her. 'We'll only be there a little while and then we're coming home.'

'I don't feel well.'

'We'll barely be a couple of hours.'

'Just go without me. Why do you need me there?'

'Oh, forget it,' Mum says, taking her jacket off.

'Why?' I follow her. 'Just go without me. Why can't you just go?'

'I don't know what the bloody point is. All week we've done sod-all and now we can't even do this.' I see her throw her jacket onto her bed before she slams her bedroom door. I go back into my room, push my palms into my eyes.

Dad's at the door again. 'This is the first time off your mother's had since Christmas. This week we were meant to go away on holiday but that had to be cancelled. All she wants is a trip out as a family. *Two hours* and you can't give her that. All the hard work she does every day and you can't do two hours and go half an hour down the road with us.' He waits for an answer I don't have, then slams my door.

I go to my window and look out to the right. In the distance, I can see as far east as The Deep and the ships docked at Hull. Come on, I can nearly *see* Spurn Point. I can make it there. But the thoughts hit me again and reduce me into my chair. Come on, come on. The footsteps and angry voices are all over the house, up and down the stairs. I don't know where my brothers are. I hear Mum open her bedroom door and go downstairs. More voices. Maybe this is it, they're getting ready to leave without me. I open my laptop and pretend to work. Dad pushes my door open. He slams my laptop shut, picks it up and throws it. It snags on its power cord, which pulls taut and knocks a speaker, but pulls free, hits the wall and falls onto my bed.

'What're you doing?' I demand, pushing my chair back out his way.

He grabs the speakers, yanks their wires until the plug under the table comes loose, grabs my Xbox, rips all the connections out the back, throws it all out my door. Gets hold of my monitor. The power cable comes free but the video cable is screwed in, which he doesn't realise. He rips, rips, rips the monitor until the cable breaks from the socket, throws it out my door. Grabs any controller and remote on my desk, reaches under the desk and gets all the wires he can in his hands. Whatever he's shouting, I can't hear. I say something, or maybe I don't. The door slams again. I sit in silence. He's *confiscating* things? I'm seventeen. I bought all of this myself. The door opens again.

'How much do I owe you?' Dad says.

'What?'

'How much do I need to pay you for last week, so we're square?'

I don't answer, or look up.

'*How much?*'

'Two hundred.'

'Right,' he says, goes downstairs. Under my feet, I feel the front door slam. His car starts and fades down the street. I stay where he left me, not knowing what to do, or what's just happened. I think about Spurn Point, how ridiculous it is that I can't go, even now, whilst the flurry of images are still behind my eyes, how out of control everyone is, that everyone is against me.

There's a dint in the wall. I pick my laptop up and check for damage. Brush blue powder from the wall off its corner. There's a scuff but that's all. Snagging on the power cord saved it from smashing completely. Or maybe Dad hesitated mid-throw.

The front door opens and the footsteps come up the stairs. Again I brace myself. Dad takes out his wallet, pulls a wad of money out, counts it, hands it to me.

'There. We're settled. I never want to see you there again.'

I take the money from his hand.

Dad leaves the house again, the front door slams, the car engine starts and fades away. I fold the money and put it on the table, where a few wires remain. Quietly close my door. Then for the first time since I was six, I burst into tears.

I try not to make any noise. My jaw shudders and I need to sniff. I pray James and Jordan don't come in. I sit on the corner of my bed. My tears make small pats on the covers between my legs. My nose runs and I've got no choice but to sniff, so I pretend to clear my throat after.

The door opens again. Mum sits next to me.

After a minute she says, 'Don't cry. Hey?'

'Everything's fucked,' I say.

'Well...'

I sneak to the bathroom, blow my nose into a tissue and flush the chain. *Look at you*, I think, looking into my blotchy eyes in the mirror, *you're crying*.

44

Summer creeps under me. At home it's back to silent meal times and staying out of my parents' way.

Mum speaks to me, but isn't over my refusal to go to Spurn Point. Me and Dad settle into another phase of not speaking. I'm still stunned by his reaction. It's re-awoken how furious I used to feel with him. Storming into my room, breaking my possessions, ripping wires. I should have sworn and shouted, maybe tried to overpower him, gone and broken some of *his* shit. The urge was there at the time, and I might even be capable, but I was too frightened. Not just of him, but of causing more hatred than there already is wedged between us. Of going past a point we can't come back from. But why should I be the one who cares about that? He clearly doesn't.

Jordan's the only one I want to hang out with. I don't know if he doesn't notice the rifts growing between everyone or if he's far wiser than I give him credit for and chooses to be completely neutral, but he never seems to care what's going on. When I take my bedroom electronics back, like a reprimanded toddler asking for his fucking toys, me and Jordan play the World War II shooter *Call of Duty 3* online together for long hours. If you get shot, your character falls to the floor and you can shout for the help of another team member to heal you before you die completely. As you bash away at the "help me" button, your character nonchalantly says 'Medic!' like his gaping wounds are a minor inconvenience he could do with a hand sorting out. And you often watch as your teammates completely ignore your calls for help. When dozens of fallen soldiers litter the streets, and they're all muttering 'Medic!', it's pretty disturbing.

Me and Jordan chat aimlessly, staring at the screen. We do impressions of the things they say on the game. I mention looking forward to going back to Leggott next week, because part of me is.

Dad comes in for the first time in a fortnight. He looks at the screen, then to me. And as always it makes me ashamed of whatever I'm doing.

'Are you busy tomorrow?'

'Why?'

'We've got a job in Beretun Green and your uncle Harvey needs help lifting the units in. There's no one else to help him.'

'Okay,' I say, before I get chance to think, or muster the courage to say no.

He leaves.

I thought you never want to see me there again, I should've said. But I know he wouldn't have asked unless he was really desperate. I don't know much about what's happened at work since I got fired but Dad's busier and stretched thinner than ever. From what little I see of him, he appears both energised and exhausted by it.

I spend the rest of the day lost in a kind of nightmare about tomorrow.

When morning arrives, I get up early and put my work clothes on but feel a foaming sickness. I nibble my breakfast and Dad says, 'Ready?'

'I don't think I'm coming,' I say. Remembering how ill I felt last time I worked with Harvey mixes with images of what might happen this time. I'm frozen to the spot like I was before Spurn Point.

Dad stares at me, his hand on the back door handle.

He opens it and steps out.

Steps back in.

'*Please?*'

'I can't.'

45

The Hummer doesn't have the boot space to move James out, and my parents are worried whether it can make the drive to Nottingham. So we load up Mum and Granddad's cars. Mum follows James about, giving him worried instructions whilst we pack. James smiles and puts an arm round her. Jordan watches in his hand-me-down black vest with a silver eagle on it. When we're done I give James a last hug. He and Mum climb into one Fiesta, Dad waits in the other. As they pull away and James spots me out the driver's window, I flip him the middle finger; he grins and does it back.

It takes a couple of hours to move into James's room, which is substantially larger than mine. I stick up the Radiohead cover art I printed out and the photos from school. James has left a few bits of memorabilia behind – photos of his friends wedged into the frame of his surfboard mirror, half ripped-off stickers on the drawers, a rolled newspaper – I don't move these things. Jordan stands by the door and asks what I'm doing, even though he can see what I'm doing. Since I don't want his help, he plays Xbox and I work around him.

'There!' I finally say.

It's September.

I go back to the workshop despite my disdain of Dad. A bloke arrives on Monday morning and puts a Liverpool FC sports bag down, comes up to me and extends a hand. 'Now, mate. I'm Elliot. Your old man's said I can work here.' He's known Dad since he was nineteen, when Dad employed him to work at Bright-Spec Windows.

I slop tar-like paint onto metal bars we then fix over the windows and doors of the workshop. I weld sashes, chip out the burn-off with a hammer and chisel, drill out drainage slots, sweep the floors, check the time, keep away from Dad. Elliot works at his trestles and has the odd polite chat with me. 'Felt like a long one today, mate,' he says. I feel sorry that he's only got me to talk to, after the bustling workshop of lads he's come from.

Working here forces me to have dirty hands. At home I wash them all the time, particularly before eating. But here it's like some healthy muck can't hurt. I eat a pack of crisps with slightly blackened fingertips, feeling like a proper man. When Nanna sees me, she comments on how "well" I look. 'You've got colour in your cheeks, boy. Hasn't he?' She turns to Dad.

'Yeah,' he says.

A second email from Sophia: *You are an ostrich!* it opens. *I get that you don't want to be in touch anymore, but to email me once and have me think we're on the mend, only to not respond afterwards, that's just sadistic.* I fetch the old dictionary from the top of the piano and look up "sadistic", though I already get the gist.

The day before college reopens, I watch *Saving Private Ryan*, in the hopes that it will put my nerves into perspective. In the evening I'm invited to play *Gears of War* at Morgan's with a big bunch of mates, but I'm worried I'll catch an illness there. Morgan had a stomach bug about eight months ago; it might still be lingering on his breath, his skin, between the cushions of his sofa, amongst the dust on the floor. But they need a second copy of the game, so I walk down there to give them mine without entering the house, holding my breath as I hand it over.

I play 'Be Here Now' by Ray LaMontagne on my iPod and enjoy the wind and the darkness. Maybe things'll turn out okay. If I concentrate on the passing of time, the thirteen hours between now and getting on the bus tomorrow morning can seem as long as two weeks.

I heard that last year a tiny nerd from school was waiting for the bus with everyone else on the first day of Leggott, before announcing, 'You know what? No.' He turned round and walked off, scrapping the idea of going to college altogether. Did he feel nervous about it, like I do?

And then there's Morgan. He went to Lindsey, down the road from Leggott, for a few months. One night, so he says, and it's hardly the sort of thing you'd lie about, he got off the bus and needed a shit so bad he knew he couldn't wait until he walked home so he shat in the nearest row of conifers. A while after, Morgan dropped out of college. And I wonder if there's a connection. Probably not.

But I still avoid those conifers.

It's the first morning of term. I cross Ferriby Road and climb the fence into Top Field.

Did I ever plan to go? I wonder, pushing down a wiry branch and stepping over it on the trail down into the trees.

Yes. It was all I wanted.

Can I go back and ask Mum to take me into college, since I can't face the bus?

No.

There's a massive STOP sign lying over the long grass we hid in last month, playing Trackers. How the hell did it get down here? I put my foot under its edge and lift it up. And bugger me. Three or four mice scatter outwards and disappear.

With a piece of glass I scrape a marking into the smooth trunk of a tree.

A couple of women walking their dogs head my way. I chuck the glass into the weeds and check my hand isn't cut.

'Morning,' I say.

'Morning!'

The dogs pant happily and run past me.

Out the other side of Tree Field, I tread between the thick wads of grass that can twist an ankle, the low bramble creepers and the nettles below Death Hill. The plants lick my trousers and my legs soon feel the damp denim. I lean on one of the only sections of picket fence still standing and watch the workmen dig foundations. What was a large pile of mud is now a small hill; a digger reverses up its slope and tips another load on top.

No one's home when I get back. I load *Oblivion* into my Xbox and start a new game. I don't want to play this, but there's nothing else to do. I keep the volume low, in case I hear anyone arrive. Which happens ten minutes later. There's just enough time to turn off the Xbox and open my backpack like I'm getting work out before Dad reaches the landing.

'You didn't go, then,' he says at the door.

I shake my head.

He sighs. But for once it's not an angry or disappointed sigh. I don't know what it is. He backs out and goes downstairs. I sit still and listen to him make a sandwich, eat it watching TV, put his pots away, head back out for work.

At five I meet Emma at the bus stop. She steps off with her binder under her arm and a big smile. We walk up to Top Field, look for a patch of grass we're sure doesn't have dog shit on and sit down. Emma tells me about her day. She does this whether I ask her or not, and I love it. A story about any girl who looked at her funny, every person who put their hand up in class, the work she's been set, what I missed in the Maggy May. I pick a flattened dandelion leaf and tear it either side of the stem. It's turning into a pleasant evening. The sun's setting just noticeably earlier than a few weeks ago. I feel like once I make it to October, when it's dark for the bus ride home, I'll be able to go to college. But I can't just take a month off.

'I keep thinking about this idea of a year off,' I say.

'Yeah? But we're back around to the start of term again.'

'It doesn't matter. I've not paid my bus fees yet.'

'What will you do?'

'Work at my dad's for a year. Pick things back up next September.'

Emma repositions her bag and lies back on it, links her fingers over her stomach. Looks up at the sky.

'Will you stay with me?' I ask.

'Why wouldn't I?'

'I'll be a year behind you. You'll be moving on to uni and I'll be stuck here.'

'That doesn't matter to me.'

46

My vision throbs. The gaggle of passengers' mouths move as though on sped-up film; behind them, the hedgerows rush past on the meandering road overlooking Scunthorpe. I feel the flush of imminent vomiting.

I crunch Polos and swallow the minty grit on my walk over the courtyard to Tutorial. Friends joke that eating too many Polos will give me the shits, but it's not true. It's sugar-free things that do that, like chewing gum. I've read the small print warning labels.

This little shelter by the pond used to emit a thin tobacco scent that hung in the cold air and comforted me, but you can't smoke here anymore.

'I'm here to support you if there's a problem with your studies. If it's getting to be overwhelming for you, or if you don't feel your lessons are bringing the best out of you,' our new personal tutor Neil says. 'But also if there's anything you need support with confidentially. Even if you're sure I can't help you, I'll put you in touch with the right person who can.'

"Trampers" is a dead end running alongside one of the sports fields. Big willow trees on one side, houses on the other. I can't spot the tramp that usually haunts the place, but there is the Mary's Ice Cream truck; it's common knowledge that the scratty guy serving the goods is a paedophile. He's trying to squeeze some business out the students lounging on the field on these last days of summer.

I duck under the dangling willow twigs and sit on the grass, take out my Steinbeck novel. Put it back in my bag. Go home.

I place my cup of tea atop a pile of music books on the lid of the piano and sit down. Ribbon and metal bolts fasten a floral-patterned carpet material to the wobbly piano stool beneath me. It came from the alcoholic neighbour we had at our old house, who's dead now. The ribbon tears when I try to get a finger under it, and a wisp of grey smokes out the split. Smell the seat and the dust seems to latch onto the skin and hair of your nostrils. You can open it to reveal more music books, old cornet mouthpieces, the two recorders me and James played in primary school, four ostrich feathers. Residual traces of saliva must still be on the mouthpieces and recorder beaks. Childhood saliva. I think about the stool's dust kind of osmosing into my jeans, into my underwear, into me. Our old neighbour's house essence, that worked its way into the fabric, now works its way back outwards, into our house, like fine spores.

Jesus, the man's dead, and he was kind. Show some respect.

I open the piano and play that opening jingle of 'The Entertainer' a dozen times – the only song I really know. Then I download and print off the sheet music for Radiohead's 'Like Spinning Plates' and make an inroad to learning it, barely stringing two notes together. My right hand begins the looping melody. Slow and stumbling, my head looking up and down from the music to the keys. I learn the first two bars and try to introduce the left hand's part, but it's too hard.

It'll soon be the weekend.

47

Emma wants us to go to Ben's together, but I tell her to meet me there and walk down on my own. He's moved house. His parents have given him the bedroom above the garage, separate from the house, with a little kitchen and bathroom downstairs. It's like he has his own place. I smoke a cigar outside at the patio table and sip on thirteen-pence lemonade.

Emma arrives; she puts her hands on my shoulders and kisses my cheek.

'You stink,' she says.

'Thanks!'

She giggles, hugs a friend, goes inside.

George arrives with another older boyfriend. He wears shorts and a cap, has thick hairy calves, earphones hung round his neck. He joins me, Ant and Morgan at the patio table and tells us about the time he had sex in a sauna and almost fainted, but on the upside, 'Sweat makes a right lube.' Ant cackles which makes it hard not to laugh. I take the communal Southern Comfort and add some to my lemonade.

We play drinking games on the floor of Ben's room. I lean against the Warhammer desk. Holly's beside me. 'I practically live here now,' she says, looking through her hand of cards. 'It's only a couple nights a week I sleep at home.'

I look at Emma, sat against the bed, leaning over a box of cheesy chips; she tucks her hair behind an ear with one hand, stabs the chips with a plastic fork with the other.

'Still thinking about a year out?' she asks on the walk home.

'No idea.'

'You've barely come in yet, this term.'

'I know.'

She falls quiet.

Another thing we've never done together: watch a film. It doesn't bother me, but it's just crossed my mind.

We pass the trodden-flat flowerbeds and low white fence surrounding The Carnival's car park. I squatted down there beside

Tommy nearly three years ago and threw up between my feet: beer and Red Bull. Then he was sick too. We laughed whilst it slowly streamed down the path, around our feet, off the kerb. The dull thump of the gig behind us. I grabbed my drink and stood up to head back inside.

Why didn't it matter back then? Because I was drunk? Because I was only a five-minute walk from home? The act of being sick isn't what bothers me. It's distance and time that's the problem. The company. The *reason*.

The Carnival's shut down, now: out of business, changing hands – whatever happens to pubs too far out in the sticks.

'Are you *sure* you're alright?' Emma asks again.

Late at night, when Emma's long-since gone, the sound of the front door opening wakes me. The quiet breath of the outside. It's Mum and Dad. I listen to their shoes scuff on the mat, before being placed under the stairs. The door gently closes. The kettle works up to the boil.

'Granddad had a fall,' Mum says the next morning.

'What, he tripped up?'

'Well… He said he was getting up from his chair and next thing he knew he was on the floor. He said his legs just gave. There's some bruising under his knee but he seems alright.'

'What's wrong with his legs?'

Mum sighs. 'Old age.'

She goes into the dining room, comes back with the clothes horse, places it by the radiator behind me. She takes her mobile out the little basket on the counter, looks at the screen, then drops her hand to her side. 'Have *you* heard from James?'

'Only in his first few days there,' I say.

'God's sake.'

'What?'

'He doesn't reply to my texts. Could be in the bottom of a ditch for all I know.' She presses a few buttons, puts the phone to her ear and walks out the kitchen.

48

In Literature, our teacher calls me over whilst the rest of the group study.

'Have you chosen a question?' He talks quietly, marking work at the same time.

'I was going to do the fourth one.'

'You haven't started yet?'

'I mean, yes. I'm doing the fourth one. Picking my own text.'

'You're meant to clear that with me before you start. You don't know that because you don't show up to any of my lessons.' He circles his pen above the paper. Jots another note. His hand is podgy, his knuckles hairy; white stubble rides the quiver of his double chin as his mouth moves. 'What are you writing on?'

'*Grapes of Wrath.*'

'Didn't the texts on the list appeal to you? Did you read them over summer?'

'Of course,' I lie, both intimidated and annoyed by the questioning.

'You got a C last year.' His fingernail finds my name on the class list and our respective grades. The nib of his pen then hovers over an empty square beside the one with a C in it. 'What are you aiming for by June?'

'At least a B.'

He puts the pen down. 'How do you expect to *improve*, let alone *match*, your AS grade when you don't attend?'

'By working really hard. And improving my attendance.'

'Have you thought about what you're doing after this year?'

'I don't know yet,' I say.

'Look around the group. Almost everyone in here is aiming to go to university. More than half are applying to study English. Look here at their predicted grades: A, A, B, A, B, B, A, A. That's why they're working so hard, why they come in.'

'I *do* work hard.'

He scrunches one eye.

Is everyone outrunning me? It's better than if I'd taken this year off. It's better than nothing.

Fucking dumpy Literature tutor.

I pull up a chair in the Maggy May and eat a few more Polos. Our table of mates are playing cards, but it's not like last year. Last year we screamed and laughed, threw our hands down like the games had real stakes, like they were a new invention. Now, everyone's just slouched behind their hands, flopping the next card down. Someone wins, scoops the cards back in and deals again without a word.

There's a double Media Studies lesson this afternoon at the top of B-Block, where you can look through the steel-framed window, over the sports field and the mobile units where I saw that guy have a fit on the floor, to see four towering conifers. I picture running down the B-Block stairs, sick pouring from my mouth, splashing on the floor and my legs, a knot of girls screaming at the sight, pressed against the wall, trying to stay away from the stinking mess. The relentless drumroll of images gets louder. I don't think I can go up there.

My molars crush another Polo. After five or six of them, sugar gathers in the recesses of my teeth and the taste gets kind of fuzzy.

'You playing, Chris?' Cartwright hits the deck of cards against the table a few times to straighten the pile into a solid block.[17]

'Nah, I've got to be somewhere,' I say, calmly as can be. And then I go home.

49

No one's here. I sit a cup of tea on the top of the music books, scooch my legs under the piano and study the sheet music for 'Like Spinning Plates'.

---

[17] Everyone will pile into here when it's lunch. It will be even more crammed than now. It's getting towards the end of September – the sun's *still* out on the journey home. Emma will be on the bus, right next to me.

The letter box goes *flump* and a light object hits the doormat. I already know it's Jordan's pre-ordered copy of *Halo 3*. He's not home for a few hours yet so I try to forget it's there waiting to be played. Besides, video games are surely a treat you earn after arriving home from college having done a full day. If I go on my Xbox when I'm not at college, watch porn and wank once or twice, it's not *earned* fun. It's lethargic. Filling the hours.

When Jordan comes home at four, he'll often be the first person I've spoken to since waking up; I catch myself following him around and chatting whilst he makes a coffee. A dog that's been left alone all day.

'Like Spinning Plates' is a single-bar loop that shifts chords, up and down the keyboard. You move your fingers in a similar order but in different places. That's tricky enough, but it's the notes that seamlessly glue one chord to the next that get me. Every note of the left and right hands alternate, never pressing a key at the same time; two melodies that plait into each other. I play super slow, making cock-up after cock-up.

I heat a tin of soup and eat it with five slices of bread. Walk down to the gym to do some chest and triceps on my own.

The pond that formed in the little car park during the floods has long since dried up, leaving behind a dusting of black silt between the ridges of concrete.

50

The man who lies on the low wall of Barton's mental home hocks a glob of phlegm into the semicircle of fag ends on the pavement before him. From under the folds of his coats or the nooks of his body, a mature smell with a faint sour spike reaches across the space between us and finds my nostrils. I cross the road and wonder how I might now be infected and when the symptoms will begin.

The sun emerges over the terraces; it's going to be another warm day.

At the far side of the subway, two railings are positioned in such a way to stop motorbikes passing through. It doesn't work. Crossers come through here all the time; it's the quickest, out-of-sight way to the quarry. Me and James once used a stick to paste ochre dog shit onto the railings. We sat up there on the concrete arch, giggling and spluttering when a guy on a crosser placed his hands on our spread to balance his bike. A bloke walked through shortly after.

'You won't be laughing when I chuck you off that fucking wall,' he shouted up to us, gripping one of the bars in anger.

'We aren't laughing at you,' I lied.

Years later, I still suck my stomach in and hold my bag up as I step between the railings. The road thins and I can see down to the Humber.

Guess where I am, I text Ben. *Walkin past quarry. Suns out, all alone.*

And I'm packt like a sardine on the bus. Need those grades tho.

Not the envious reply I wanted.

Everyone's moving forward. What a failure I'll be if I end up having to retake this year. It makes me need to walk faster, but what use is that? I'm falling behind either way.

A track forks off the road, under a tunnel of whatever thorny plant grows the hard, red berries Dad would sneakily throw at the back of my head as a child. To my left, a broken picket fence before the sheer drop into the quarry below. I lean over and feel an urge to tip further. Two bikers speed over the flint and chalk mounds in the basin, the angry buzz of their engines a distant muddle of echoes. Rumour has it, a kid once got in a tractor tyre and rolled down one of the near-vertical sides. Surely that would've killed him.

The trail follows a gentle slope until it meets the shore of the river. I grab handfuls of grass to guide me down the clay cliff onto the shingles. Over the muddy bay, behind the block structures and conveyor belts of the cement works, steam snakes from the hundred-metre chimney, then hangs almost completely still in the air.

A movement in my abdomen grabs my attention. I stand evaluating myself for a moment. Do I need a shit, suddenly? This far from home?

I set off walking back towards Barton.

Why have I come all this way on foot? Nearly to South Ferriby. How is this any better than college? The walk from here to home is nearly as long as the bus ride! Faster, faster. My hands almost look for the drug pocket. But don't. And don't run, either. If I take tablets or break into a run, it'll be confirmation that I'm desperate and ill. Just walk like everything's okay.

The base of the Humber Bridge's south tower is back in view. I clamber over a peninsula of chalk boulders and old wooden stilts, and within minutes I'm on familiar ground. Far from home, but at least familiar. Whatever was happening in my stomach has stopped. I fill my cheeks and blow out. Don't stop marching, though; it's still a long way home.

51

Mum drives me to Leggott, and on the dual carriageway she looks up at the sky and remarks that it's an "Indian Summer", which makes me uneasy. India means heat, germs, spicy food; summer means burning light, long days and high visibility.

'Oh, listen. I like this song,' she says, hesitantly turning her stereo up a single notch. It's that fucking "beautiful girl, you got me suicidal" song. The way he yaps the third syllable of the word "suicidal" sounds like ripples of heat rising from a road, the temple throb of a head squeezed in a migraine.

I open my mouth to say 'I hate it' but don't bother.

Mum talks away whilst I watch the traffic lights we stopped at before the uni evening when I thought I'd shit myself.

Keep it together. The light's green already, look. The tablets are here.

I pinch the skin on the front of my neck: it's too tight a fit. Flattening my oesophagus.

Sugary smells and tastes haunt my mouth and throat. Classic bars. Caramel Rockys. Pots of creamy rice pudding with jam swirled in.

Caramel stirred into a yoghurt. Chocolate baubles. Banana. Strong coffee. A scoop of clotted cream. The slowly thinning dribble of treacle from a sticky tin. Powdered icing on rich cake. Just mash it all up until it's a bucket's worth of confectionery slop that in this daydream I can't stop spooning into my gob.

52

October arrives.

Dad leaves for work. Jordan makes toast and spreads peanut butter, jam and Bovril onto the slices and presses them together into a sandwich. Mum asks if I've heard from James, I say no.

Sat on the fence overlooking the giant mud mound, I listen through the new Radiohead album, *In Rainbows*. A JCB crawls between the foundations where builders lay breezeblock walls. The sun: it's a little lower in the sky at this time of day than it was when term started. Rising later. Can we call this autumn yet?

I walk through an old quarter of Barton, past high brick walls, bent in age like they've grown bellies. Behind iron gates, long drives stretch back into conifers. Creepers cling onto everything. Towering bay windows on Victorian terraces, with wooden frames and cloudy single panes, peels of paint fallen down onto the front yards below, where grass sprouts through pebbles and dead cars corrode. Our old athletics team would come here to do running drills in the dark.

By ten I get home. Play piano. Write college assignments. Watch porn. Play Xbox. Rub my eyes. It's two o'clock. Go downstairs and turn the TV on. There's a new channel called Dave that plays old episodes of *Top Gear* all the time. My Nanna pulls up to drop off whatever meat she's bought at Scunthorpe market. I tell her it's an "early day" for me. She opens the meat packaging and tells me to smell it, looking at my face for an awed reaction. What's good raw pork *meant* to smell like? Emma comes over later on. I feel lethargic from being cooped all day. 'I've got work to do later,' I tell her.

She sighs.

'What?' I say.

'Nothing.'

'Then can you stop doing that? I get sighed at enough by my dad.'

I think back to spring when she asked, 'Are you getting tired of me?' I couldn't say it: the answer was yes. I'd even told Ant there's "something I want to talk about" but couldn't admit to anyone that I was seeing an end to Emma and me. That was, what, five or six months back, though. Things have changed. We're stronger than ever.

She stands on her tiptoes at the front door and kisses me. Then again. And again. I force a giggle. My eyes focus past Emma's head, to the lights of her mum's car, waiting by the road.

* * *

The sun flashes between the trees when we leave Winterton, then between the terraces in Scunthorpe. I eat another polo. Skull Lady gets off in town centre. Over the square, I see someone with a drooping sausage roll in a Greggs wrapper. He takes a bite and it's too hot: he chews in open-mouthed snaps and little plumes of steam come out. I close my eyes. The bus carries on to college.

After barely a minute in the Maggy May I turn heel and hurry back towards town. Nine Inch Nails' *Year Zero* plays in my ears. A mist has settled over the streets; I make little smiles with my cheeks and feel them stiffening.

I'm writing an essay when I hear the door unlock downstairs. It's Dad.

Listen. That's his shoes tapping on the hollow kitchen floor, the fridge opening and shutting, clingfilm being peeled off a bowl of cold leftovers, the leather of the living room chair scrunching under his weight, the TV turning on. Channels changing. His fork hitting and scraping on crockery.

I stay absolutely still. This computer chair is prone to clunk about in its stand if I put too much weight on one arse cheek. I get up slow enough to make my thighs ache, take *The Great Gatsby*, lower myself onto the carpet and lie flat.

This happens a few times. Dad comes home for lunch and usually knows if I'm here. But if he doesn't, I try to keep it that way, which in a thin-walled house isn't easy. He shouts, 'Hello?' and I risk not answering; my earphones are kept within reach, ready to jam in and use as an excuse for not hearing his call if he comes upstairs.

His lunch is at twelve-thirty, so I get ready: lying on the floor with a book to read. But the back-door handle can sometimes chop down at half ten or two o'clock and startle me. So I learn to keep silent at all times, to hear cars stopping and turning their engines off. I peek through the curtains to see if it's him, again and again.

53

I haven't made it through one full day of college this term. I'm afraid to open my emails – none of them are good news:
It's time to make a choice.
You must address this.

One afternoon on the bus home, Emma's beside me. She goes into her bag, pulls out a wad of printouts and hands them over.

'I was talking to Mum about what's going on with you,' she says. *Anxiety/Panic*, the leaflets are titled, with a stick figure of a person with frizzy hair holding their head and frowning. 'She thinks it might be this.'

'Right...' I leaf through them. Large fonts, bullet points. 'You've been talking to your mum about me?'

'We talk about everything. We're best friends,' Emma says to her knees, her shoulders held up in a shrug.

I put the papers away.

'Will you look through them?'

'Sure.'

'Sorry,' she says. 'I didn't say it was *you*, really. I just said like, "What would you recommend to someone who acts this way?" It's her job to help people like this.'

'She'll put two and two together, though, considering she knows I miss a lot of college. Won't she?'

'Sorry.'

54

'Head!' Mum warns, putting her hand on Granddad's scalp and bending him into the passenger seat of her Fiesta like she's gently arresting him. He puts his belt on and rests the end of his ancient cane between his shoes.

'Very good,' he says. It's the first time Granddad's left the house in ages. He's wearing a black blazer with what look like strange medals on his breast.

We're not allowed to ask him about the war.

Mum drives us up to our house. Granddad shuffles through the front door, one hand on his cane, the other palming at the frame for something to hold onto. Mum walks closely behind. I've only seen Granddad run once, a good twelve years ago, when Jordan was crawling over the edge of The Ditch. It looked laboured. He's a very still person. And in the still years since he ran those eight or ten steps over the grass, I think the ability to do any more than shuffle has left him.

Even when they aren't here, Mum prepares food for my grandparents as much as possible, cooking tea for six mouths, stretching clingfilm over a tray and driving down to feed her parents.

I set the dining room table and we eat chicken, gravy, vegetables. Granddad asks Jordan and me in turn, 'And what is happening in your education?' I'm good at talking away about a life at college that doesn't really exist. Jordan dutifully says, 'Good, thanks,' and then frowns when Mum taps his shin with her foot under the table.

Granddad must think school and college are way better than they really are. As though kids still respect their teachers. I'd hate for him to know what they're really like, and what I'm really like. His class was taught how to ring church bells in their free time for Christ's sake.

Today's the last Sunday of half term. I help Dad wash up whilst making Jordan laugh. Make a row of teas and hand them out. Nanna arrives, who by the time I come into the living room has got the old folks comparing the medicines they take, for the blood pressures that are too high or too low, the cholesterol levels that are at a number which means nothing to me, bones complaining, digestive systems going haywire, epilepsy or stroke prevention, post-heart bypass medication, post-bowel surgery medication.

Nanna sits forward. 'I've got one of them trays that divide your doses. I take three in the morning, soon as I wake up. Then two at eleven, two at two. I take five, twenty minutes before me tea in the evening. Then three before bed.'

'And do you get any of these "side effects"?' asks Granddad.

'Well, I get *diarrhoea* now and then,' she says, really emphasizing that word.

'Mmm,' says Granddad.

I'm pretty sure he's like me, and would rather not review bodily functions.

Nanna, she doesn't give a shit. In fact she enjoys listing whatever she's going through.

I go upstairs and play *Halo 3*.

There's something unsettling about Sundays. Knowing it's college tomorrow, of course, but also the sluggishness. The big dinner, feeling my stomach heavy and full, the smell of food throughout the house from morning until night. My grandparents coming up. Their slow, tame conversation. The house being so quiet despite being full. Like a wake. Having to keep all the windows closed and the heating on for their thin blood. I know Mum is secretly hoping they leave soon because she has a mountain of notes to write before work tomorrow – she'll be up working until the early hours. It's hard to put a finger on why, but it all makes me feel like something's wrong.

Jordan comes in and he's like an escape, a window being opened. He watches me shoot things and we don't say a word. To the side of my drawers, that rolled newspaper James left behind has turned a little yellow.

If we're lucky, James will take the train up from Nottingham. I hug him when he comes through the door and think how strange it is that my brother now smells of a foreign home. James has this manner where he always looks a bit sad even when he's happy; but even knowing this, I do look at his face and wonder whether he wants to be here at all. After lunch, Dad will wash the pots up and offer to drive him back to uni, a five-hour round trip on the only afternoon of the week Dad isn't working his bollocks off.

* * *

'One month to go!' says Emma. 'Our one-year anniversary.'

'Well, *technically*,' I reach over to the swivel chair, find my phone in my jeans pocket and check the time, 'it's one month minus about four hours. We got together on the way back from college, just as we were between Ferriby and Barton, so it would've been quarter to five-ish.'

I'm lying on my front, propped up on elbows.

Emma retreats beneath her covers and pulls them up so only her face sticks out, smiling.

It makes me laugh, which immediately makes Emma laugh too. God, her face is nice. I lean over and kiss her.

'What?' she says. 'What?'

My lips touch her teeth.

'You're just funny,' I say.

'I love when I make you laugh. I never feel like I can make you laugh.'

'I laugh *at* you enough.'

'Gee, thanks.'

'Can I open the window?'

'Noooo,' she says, but I get up anyway. Lift the latch and push the window out. The living room below us throws a little light onto the white pebble yard, the stack of plastic chairs and a table, the shed and bins. Beyond the back fence, it's too dark to see the field and the abandoned tractor. Cars quietly *shwoosh* by somewhere I can't see. The cool air touches my body.

'How can you be hot? It's freezing!'

'I must've done all the work,' I say.

Emma tilts her head forward with raised eyebrows.

I pull my boxers on and sit at the foot of the bed. This is the first time I've been to Emma's in weeks. She always comes to me nowadays, and that's difficult enough.

'What if I don't make it on our anniversary? What if I can't see you?'

'Then I'll come over to your house and break in, and find you wherever you are. I'm stronger than I look. I'll drag your ass out,' Emma's head says.

I smile and hope she's joking. She promised never to come over uninvited again.

November 16th.

November 16th.

November 16th.

November 16th.

November 16th.

55

Our other Literature teacher has a mass of wavy maroon hair and thick glasses. She tips her head back and puts on a husky northern voice like the Mel B caricature in *Bo' Selecta!* and it's hard to tell whether she does it to be funny. It happens midway through any given sentence. There's no pattern. As though she keeps getting possessed. One lesson, I ask if I could have the work from last week.

'*Why* weren't you here?' she snaps.

'I was just poorly.'

Then she disappears, and the dumpy teacher has to take over her share of classes. Is she sick? Injured?

I walk past the English block towards one of the staff car parks and I see her out there, crying, distressed. A man, with the hesitation of someone who only knows her as a colleague, rests his hands on her arms, then hugs her. I skirt the car park so she doesn't know I've seen her.

'Are you like me?' I mouth.

56

The clocks have changed.

Grass thaws under my foot. Looking back, dark prints mark my gently snaking route over Top Field. Down the slope, I touch a few frosted roots with my toes to see how slippery they are. Take a close-up picture of a frozen leaf. Squat down and flick backwards through the camera's memory card: here's a picture of dead, wet leaves on the ground; here's one that looks through the trees, when the leaves were still green. I look up at the autumn and turn the camera off. Walk into Tree Field. I spot the marking I made on the tree trunk. Trace my finger over it, melting a little line through the frost. The raw edges I cut into the bark have smoothed over. It's more like a scar than a cut now. Is the glass shard I used still on the floor? I swipe the grass stalks and dead weeds with my foot. Not there. Where do these things go?

The quiet jingle of collar bells approaching.

I shoulder my bag and act natural, walk down the grassy path, like I'm headed somewhere.

The two dogs trot past me without a sniff; their owners walk behind, chatting happily and quietly. 'Hi,' they breathe.

'Hey.'

There's a feeling, in my legs, that I've *got* to be at college. That everything's retreating, zooming out until it's too small to climb back into.

At home I flex my fingers, trying to get the blood flowing. I can't turn the heat on: it makes a humming noise, and if Dad comes home it will give away that someone's here. Warm my hands around a mug of tea, letting go whenever it gets too hot. Shield one hand with the other and breathe into the cocoon. But the warmth doesn't reach deep. I try to play 'Like Spinning Plates', but my fingers don't move fast enough. I splay my fingers out and play its chords.

The hours slug by. I work for a while, find more to do once I've completed what's been set. Lie on the sofa and watch TV, the world continuing outside. Emma asks if she can come over.

Can do. Im not free for long tho. Av got loadsa work t do xxxx

At 16:49 it's dark. I sit on the wall by the bus stop outside my street, watching the headlights bob over the roundabout and past me, down the hill. The bus comes into view and I feel a sour pang in my throat. I picture running to its doors and closing them, yelling, 'I've changed my mind, don't get off, don't see me,' to Emma's astonished face. It crosses the roundabout and indicates to pull over. The inside lights are on, the passengers clearly visible compared to the dark outside. Easy to identify. They look out the windows but I wonder if they can see me. The bad thing about lights on the bus is that everyone in the streets you pass can see you, clear as day. But the good thing is that the second you step off the bus, out of the light, you're almost invisible to the students on board.

This is it then: it's dark. It's dark on the bus ride home. We've arrived at the time of year it should be easy to go to college. It's autumn, no question. There are no excuses anymore. I should be there with Emma, walking between the students, down the aisle to the doors, gripping the handrails to keep from falling as the bus brakes to a halt.

The doors fold open and Emma hops down onto the pavement.

'Alright?' she beams. She comes up on her tiptoes to kiss me. I put my hands on her waist. Her coat is open and when we hug I'm half inside it with her. Her body is warm and I shiver, my skin waking up to how cold it is out here.

The streets are grey when I leave the house, past the dog walkers, through the trees. Each day is a different tour.

Stand by the rotting fence that overlooks the new houses being built and watch the workmen in their high-vis jackets and yellow hats. Jump over the dried-up concrete ditch and see whether a new chunk of furniture or torn-up bit of clothing has appeared in the mud. Squeeze down the bramble route, or clamber up Death Hill to look over Barton.

Walk Tofts Road, Bowmandale or Brigg Road; snake up and down the connecting streets to kill the time. Always worried I'll be seen.

An arms-width road leads to Spud Farm, down Piggery Hill or over Saxby Tops. Past the concrete slabs I ran away to as a thirteen-year-old, the rabbit warren bank, over the dual carriageway bridge and back into Barton.

Down to the river bank again and across the pebbled beaches, climbing on the rocks, the old pier struts and the derelict walls, finding where my brothers and me used to stash iron.

Along the chalky tracks running by the quarry to Ferriby. Past dens where tramps have slept – melted bottles, syringes, food packets, plastic bags I daren't look inside, Rizla tabs trod into the mud like maggots, trolleys, scorched ground, soiled clothing.

Text lies to Emma – why I'm not at college or can't come to her house. Cancel more plans. Hesitate to open emails from my tutors. Take photos to feel like my days are productive: the grass, the clouds, trees, a slug on the pavement, my iris, bramble vines stretching out a wire fence by a car garage, a busy crossing.

It's something.

I warm my hands and attempt 'Like Spinning Plates'. I learn to play it full speed, to a tee. Then I start altering the transitional notes between chords, turning them into little flourishes. I sing the vocals, improvise new second halves to the track – melodies that become a rhythmic mashing with the damper pedal pressed to make it all melt into a series of gigantic swirling chords. One rendition can last quarter of an hour if I really get into it. Then I keep the pedal down and listen to the echoes behind the wood slowly, slowly fading. Press my ear against the panel and it's still there, quieter than a breath. I bring in a kitchen chair, sit my laptop on it and record myself, silently cursing the computer's loud fans. Take the recording upstairs and warp it. Lace it with other sounds. Chop, reverse and pitch-shift it into a jittery mess. Stretch a tiny segment until it plays hundreds of times slower, over seven minutes of almost perceptible vibrations. I spend hours on music software, even designing a track made solely from a single click of the fingers. James left one of his guitars here, so I teach myself tunes on that, too. I master them. Overplay them. Then I'll drop my hands and think, what the fuck am I *doing*?

The leaves curl up and fall off, then rot into mulch as the days thread into weeks. Freezing, thawing, freezing, thawing. I watch it all.

Say hi to the dog walkers.

The mark on the tree darkens, softens.

Warm my hands around a mug and wonder what lesson I'm meant to be in.

Tell Mum and Dad it was an "early day" today.

Find out what work's been set and meet the deadlines. Wince to send an email. At this point, my tutors must look at the sender and think, *Who's C. Westoby?*

Each night, I resolve to go to college in spite of the sickness I know will crescendo from the minute I wake up. Each morning, I push against the blizzard of images, determined to scramble through it all this time. And I see it there: the bus stop. You're a coward, I shout internally, through the gales. You're sick because you're afraid of being sick.

But that doesn't make it less real. And *this* could be the time it's a virus taking hold of me.

How would I know the difference?

The occasional spike in bravery will be enough to get me on the bus.

I attend a lesson per fortnight. Sit there crunching on Polos. Sour, hot bile licks up my insides. Every minute is the minute before the vomiting and shitting begins.

Swallow.

Classmates give me an odd look as though I'm new.

I'm relieved when it's nearly the weekend, but then ask, *Why?* I didn't go to college this week anyway. What difference does a Saturday have, except that I don't take a walk before ending up right back here? What is a Sunday for but festering in that smog of central heating with my grandparents, worrying about Monday and every Monday to come?

Sitting in the lounge on a week day morning before college, with Jordan drinking a pint of strong coffee and dunking his way through a stack of chocolate digestives, I realise that not only is college out of the question, I'm uneasy even to go on my walk. What if I'm ill out there in the middle of Barton, twenty-odd minutes from home?[18] Like when I was way out at the beach overlooking the cement works and thought I suddenly needed a shit. What would I do? Who would see me?

It's dark now. Dark on the journey both to and from college. I turn around halfway across Top Field and wait to see the yellow-lit grid of windows trail by.

With every step, I recalculate how long it would take to briskly walk home, and to sprint home. The risk grows by the minute. Through the tree line, down the little slope, holding a bendy branch in case I slip on the mud, into Tree Field. Try not to think about being ill out here. It beats college, surely. Maybe just don't walk too far. Maybe, tomorrow, just creep under the kitchen window and hide behind the house again.

Christ, you're seventeen.

'Hey,' I say to the dog walkers.

---

[18] Less than twenty minutes if I walk quickly, but the faster I walk, the more ill I might get. The way snake venom spreads.

My cheeks sting. It's light enough to see, but over the far bank the carriageway lights are still on.

An anger makes itself known.

Were it not for Emma, I probably would be at college right now. Maybe none of this mess would've happened. Let's not forget, it was hard to go in for those first two months when I was single, but it got worse from the day we got together.

Is this her fault?

She makes it harder. Sat there on the bus waiting for me every day, not aware that she may as well be a rabid pit bull with an insatiable taste for raw bollocks for all the encouragement she gives me to get on and sit beside her.

But I've always had this thing, to a lesser degree. It maybe would've got worse without Emma. Or be the same whoever I went out with. At least Emma is patient. Many would have dumped me long ago. Many would tell their friends all about me.

What if I was still in school? Would I not be able to go there anymore either?

'Are you fucking stupid?' asked one of Sophia's friends on prom night when I revealed I couldn't ride the limo over to Hull with them.

I'm not so much tired as I am SICK of it, Emma wrote in spring.

There are times I tell Emma she's better off breaking up with me. But I know she won't. 'Don't you wish you were with someone who could do these things? Go places with you? Sleep over?' I say.

I wish I was alone.

58

I wander to the bottom of Barton, past Proudfoot and the Rope Walk, along Farrings Road[19], all the way up Gravel Pit Lane; stride over the ruts beside the road and wait in the verge for stray

---

[19] This is far enough. Don't go too far.

cars to pass, averting my eyes from the drivers. Branch left at the top. Over the massive roundabout where tramps live in the trees.

A thorny hedge skirts the top of the bank, dividing Chartdale and the Humber Bridge slip road. I notice a little wooden gate bedded within it.

"The clouds will part and the sky cracks open. And God himself will reach his fucking arm through just to push you down. Just to hold you down," Trent Reznor cries in my ears, his voice masked as though pouring his heart out through a tannoy, above a piano line and squelching bass.

I pull my iPod out and press pause.

Is this the problem? Am I being punished for listening to these lyrics? I mean, I deleted the worst track, but Nine Inch Nails' whole catalogue is infected with… unholiness. Blasphemy.

Maybe I should give it up completely.

And porn, too. Porn isn't right, I can feel it. Maybe that's causing the sickness. Some connection. I have prayed to be better, but God doesn't help. Not since the desperate prayer in Florida, waiting for the ferry. That was a card I could only play once, and it's played. I shouldn't have promised never to ask for anything again.

Why would God help me now, if I listen to songs promoting a hatred of him, and watch other people shagging?

So it's decided.

I climb up the wet grass, unhook the gate. Stoop under the thorny twigs. A thin park runs beside new houses and new roads, leading back through the estate to my house. It's twenty to ten: it should be safe to go home.

59

"Oh, what if I'm sick? Oh, what if I get diarrhoea?"' Mum snarls, doing an impression of something I've never actually said. She's behind the wheel, driving me through the last few junctions before college. 'Life's a risk, Chris. Jesus, do you know how many times I've been into work when I feel like absolute crap? Do you think I can just tell the people waiting for me, "Oooh, I'm not sure I feel that well today"?'

Mum may not know the extent of how little I go in, but she knows I miss a lot.

And then the letter comes.

Addressed to my parents in an innocent brown envelope so I couldn't know to intercept it. A formal invite for my parents to meet with the deputy head, to discuss my 5% attendance, to discuss my future there. I'm allowed in the meeting, so is my personal tutor, who I've only met once.

The deputy head of the whole fucking college.

In the kitchen. It's dark outside. On the round kettle I see my elongated reflection across the room.

Mum's still in her coat and heels. She's furious and puzzled. Dad's hands are on the counter by the sink. He looks out the window at what must be nothing at all.

'When you leave in the morning, what do you do? Do you even get on the bus?' Mum says.

'Course I do.' The house of lies has fallen down, but I'm pitching a new tent on the rubble. I can't stop. 'It's the lessons I don't go to.'

'Why? You know what, don't answer. I don't care. So, what, you just sit around doing nothing and then catch the bus back?'

I don't reply.

'If you're already there, you've *done* the hard part, surely. What's the difference between waiting all day for a bus home and going to a lesson?'

'I don't know.'

'Sounds about right,' Dad says.

'Don't just leave, Wayne.'

'Why?' He pauses at the door leading to the hall.

'We have to meet this woman.' She holds the letter up.

'He's made his choice, Jane.' He goes.

The door shuts.

Mum keeps quiet for a while, looking around, her arm propped on the back of the chair, holding the letter still. Thinking what to say.

She stares at me.

'Do you even get on that bus?'

'Yes. Most mornings.'

Her stare holds. And it's an expression I don't know.

She knows now.

'*Right.*'

She gets up. Puts her coat on the back of the chair and turns the oven on. Opens the fridge and starts taking food out.

'What's happening?'

'I've got to do dinner, haven't I?'

I sit here. Am I meant to leave? Speak?

The clamour when she slams the trays into the oven makes me flinch.

'I mean, can you blame your dad? You're just pissing it away, aren't you.' Her eyes are wide and tired. Blinking more than usual. Her head, very slightly, shakes side to side. 'After everything you achieved at school, and where you could be going. You're giving up. I can't believe it, Chris. I don't know where the hell it went wrong.'

'I can't help it.'

'Don't.'

The next morning, Mum stops me in the hall.

'What are you going to do, now? Are you actually off to the bus?'

I nod and go round her, out the front door. Pull it closed behind me harder than I should. It's dark and mizzle falls slowly. I smell wet tarmac. Down the street, to the bus stop. Luckily, no one I know waits here. My legs feel like they won't hold me up so I slouch onto the low garden wall behind me. Wet conifer wipes the back of my head. My insides are kneading. I try to swallow. My throat recoils from the invading measure of spit. It takes three dry gulps to force it down. Kinks in a hosepipe. A curling elephant's trunk. My stomach threatens to lurch it back up.

Car after car comes past, and then I see our bus climbing the hill. Jesus. I can't do this. Closer and closer. The moment has to last longer than this. I need time. A woman steps forward and puts her arm out. The bus indicates and slows down. I stay leant on the wall. The bus stops; its doors hiss open and the woman steps on. She exchanges money for a ticket. The driver barely acknowledges her.

The noise of passengers. Chatting, laughing.

I act natural, as though this one's not my bus. Look down the road, like the one I want will come any time soon. I don't look into the windows, in case Emma's looking right at me, barely two metres away.

The doors close and it grinds forward, over the roundabout.

I keep staring down the road. There are still a couple of people left here that I'm acting for. But inside, I'm holding my head.

A buzzing in my pocket. Emma must have seen me. I don't answer.

I'm shaking. Part of me knew I wouldn't be doing the long walk today, and I didn't bring a coat.

The next bus comes. The last one to Scunthorpe, with everyone else I know on board. Its doors open and a couple more get on.

Another bus arrives, headed to Hull. The last people here at the stop get on. The driver looks at me out the doors. I smile and put a hand up. No, not my bus, thanks.

And then Jordan crosses the roundabout and heads along Forkdale on his route to school. He spots me and nods.

I go home.

All the clunks of the door unlocking and opening will resound through the house. Somewhere upstairs, Mum will tense up. Maybe grit her teeth. She knows who it is. Opening the door is shouting up to Mum that I've failed.

I drop my bag in the kitchen and sit down, waiting for the fight.

Upstairs, the hairdryer turns back on. I let my head meet my palms. Water drips off my fringe.

'What's the matter?' Mum says, a few minutes later. Her voice restrains itself. It's almost formal. She puts two slices of bread in the toaster and pushes the lever down. Tops her cup of tea up with a little kettle water. Every movement faster and louder than usual.

'I couldn't get on the bus.'

'Why?'

'I didn't feel well. Still don't.'

'I'll have to take you in, then.' She turns over a jumper that's drying on the radiator. The toast pops up. I keep my head down until she takes her breakfast through to the lounge, then I tread quietly upstairs.

For ten minutes I hope she might forget me and just go to work.

'Let's go, then,' she calls from downstairs. I hear her plate and mug go in the dishwasher. The hollow clop of her shoes marching down the hall. The jingle of her keys. My mind is made up. She can't seriously think I'll come down.

'Go without me,' I say from the top of the stairs. 'I can't go.'

Down by the front door, she looks up at me. Her voice coiled and sharp, her eyes shining. 'Get your bag and let's go. I'm going to be late at this rate.'

'Then just go.'

She looks around, her head doing little shakes.

'I *can't*, Mum.'

The snap I was waiting for. Her voice raises: 'Then get changed and get your arse down to that workshop, and at least make a living for yourself if you're throwing your education away.'

I don't reply.

Her voice cracks into a high-pitched shout, through pressed teeth. 'I'm *wild!*'

What an odd thing to say.

She comes storming up the stairs. I move out the way.

'I've got one son who avoids me and another who's *deceptive.*'

She does something in her room and then runs past me, down the stairs again. She's still shouting as she picks her bag up and makes for the door, but it's the slight muffle through gritted teeth and the wobble in her voice I hear more than the words. The door *bangs* in its frame. Through the obscured glass, her Fiesta's little engine revs like a boy racer's car as it reverses out the drive.

I sit on the stairs for a long time.

What do I do? What the fuck do I do?

60

November 16th. Emma goes to college. I don't remember the last time I went in on a Friday. Mum and Dad know what I do, so why keep up this act of leaving only to walk around for a few hours?

My abstinence from porn and Nine Inch Nails hasn't changed how things are. Perhaps it's like the various acne medications the doctor gives me, where it takes six to eight weeks to take effect.

'Morning,' breathe the dog walkers. The dogs run past me.

The sun first peeks over the construction site. An hour later, they turn off the spotlights. In the concrete ditch is a children's toy pram, *inside* a real pram. The fabric of the canopy is punctured and turning green.

My phone buzzes.

Happy anniversary baby!! Love u lots and lots and lots! Cant wait to see u 2nit and hold u and give u ur prezzy! What u doin 2day? xxxxxxxxxxxxxxxxxxxxx

With cold thumbs I slowly concoct a similar reply.

Before the subway, turn left and through the bollards into the bottom of Chartdale. To my right is the little park beside the slip road trees. Some of the bushes have clung onto their leaves. I remember walking down to Morgan's to drop off my copy of *Gears of War* on the last day of summer. It was dark, Ray LaMontagne played in my ears, the bushes and young trees were thick with leaves that fluttered on the ends of thin branches in the warm wind. And I thought, there's a good place to hide, should I need to.

Winter has the benefits of short days and the cover of night. Summer is worse but grows thick shrubbery to hide in.

What is Emma doing right now at college? Thinking about tonight? Deep in concentration in a lesson? I picture her little frame pootling through the corridors, hugging her binder. Chatting with our group of friends, trying too hard to fit in, like she does.

At home I do a few laps around 'Like Spinning Plates', improvise for a while, sit and inspect the cracks in the piano stool's frame and think about dust. About limescale in our hard water. About tonight. Being ill at Emma's. But at least if I go there, rather than her coming here, I can leave when I want. Even if there's no one to take me home, I could leap out the door, or even a window, and disappear into the dark. Yes, it'll be pitch dark. I could even get myself over that barbed steel fence on the green outside her house and into the fields, away from any streetlights. If I get cut up, that's still better than being seen.

I do some college work and watch the oven clock creep closer to the evening. Replaying what Emma said she'd do if I couldn't go. 'I'll come over to your house… I'll drag your ass out.' She wouldn't dare. Right? Every night, I worry she'll show up at the door with her little knock, nervously hoping I'm happy to see her.

Dad drives me to Barrow. We pull into Emma's square at ten past seven. Her kitchen light's on. Nervousness tickles behind my knees and in my abdomen. I ask Dad to pick me up in one hour fifty minutes.

Emma gives me a long kiss at the door. Hugs me around the neck and says, 'Happy Anniversary!' I hear the football on and smell her dad's roll-up cigarette smoke. I'm led through to the lounge, where I say hi to her family. Emma adjusts the old throw on one of the couches and we sit down. We watch TV for a while. Emma leans into me, occasionally rocking her shoulders, trying to nuzzle ever deeper under my arm. I laugh and rub her leg, and that's when I feel the bump of a strap and buckle of suspenders under her jeans. My heart beats faster. But also, I think how I don't want to be obliged to have sex. The lingerie does oblige me. What if I become unwell *whilst we're doing stuff?* How quickly could I jump into my clothes and run out the door? How much would it hurt Emma? I look around the lounge at her parents and big sister. The room is hot. The house is hot.

'Want a cuppa?' Emma's mum says.

'Not just now, thanks.'

'I'll show you your present,' Emma says, getting up.

'I don't want to hear,' her dad laughs, and her mum giggles too.

'An *actual* present, Dad. A thing you can hold.'

'Oh, enough!' He waves his hands at us.

'Put the shovel down,' her mum says.

We go to Emma's room. I pick up the gift bag I left by the shoe rack.

'And keep your door open,' her dad shouts up the stairs, and laughs with his wife.

'Sorry about that.' Emma smiles, closing the door behind her.

I sit on her bed.

'This is for you,' I say, pulling a wrapped box and card from the bag. I've bought her a necklace, using most of the money I've got. Which is about seventy quid. She seems to love it. The card is full of romantic writing.

She gives me a card and what feels like a game or DVD.

'Open the present first,' she says. 'The card talks about it.'

I read the tag and tear the paper. It's a blank DVD case. I open it up and there's a blank disc labelled with marker pen, "Chris and Emma: 1 year together" and covered with kisses.

'Ah, wow,' I say.

'Open the card!'

Jesus, it's like opening a broadsheet: her neat handwriting fills every inch of the card. It examines the greatness of our relationship. How lucky Emma feels. How amazing I am. How we'll always be together. And a kiss for every day we've been together. Yes, 365 tiny kisses. And then a few more "for good measure". A small picture of a snowman. An explanation of what the disc is, although I'd already guessed.

'It's amazing.'

'Really?'

'Yeah, I love it. Thanks so much.'

We kiss. I make a mental note to get the DVD-watching over with tonight.

'There is something else I got for you. Well for me, for you.'

'I already know. I could feel it under your trousers.'

'Never thought it would be *you* feeling a bulge under *my* trousers.'

The time to leave gets close. I write a text to Dad, asking him to come an hour later. My thumb briefly hesitates over the send button. Can I do this? Yes.

Viewing it from this side, the hour is a gulf to cross. It's only the equivalent of missing one of the buses home from Scunthorpe town. Just picture poking around a few shops in these last sixty minutes. It will pass soon. Unless Dad doesn't come right on time. We might be talking seventy minutes. Could I hold vomit down for that long?

But even extending my time here, I can see the finish line. An elating sense of *I did it* is dispersing. You know when you're in the bath, and the water's gone cool, so you turn the hot tap on with your toe? The warmth touches your feet, spreads up your legs, meets your fingertips, closes round your shoulders.

'You okay?'

'Yeah.' I snap my phone shut.

This can't be enough for her. This can't be all Emma wants from a boyfriend.

The DVD is a slideshow of pictures involving Emma and me. Corny music plays. She's animated the photos to slide onto the screen and overlap each other. It tells a little story. Annotations like "Remember this?" and "Hehe!" roll over the screen. I put the disc back in its case, send a text to Emma saying how brilliant it was. Turn the Xbox on. Thank God today is over.

61

My feet slip from under me on Teletubby Hill. An elbow sinks into the soft mud under the grass and the wetness comes through my coat, touches my skin. I clamber into the ditch where Wykes was getting head off a girl a couple of summers back, until a few mates ran down to interrupt and caught an unwanted glance of his now-fabled oversized balls.

Today, the trees are bare and wiry, the floor carpeted with twigs. I shuffle a few of them around with my trainer. Find wrappers, shot glasses and broken glass amongst the dead wood. Think *fuck it* and climb up the beanpole trunk of a tree. Hands and feet latched onto the smooth bark, passing my weight from arms to legs, until I'm high enough to feel it wanting to bend.

On a long lap round Westfield Road I play Nine Inch Nails, since *not* listening to them wasn't getting me far. 'Every Day is Exactly the Same' is invigorating to come back to, but an unease takes its time to lift.

At home I open my laptop and think for a while; its internal fan turns on then stops, turns on then stops, turns on then kicks up to full blast. I open Firefox and type "hardcore porn" into Yahoo. I don't risk using Google, in case it remembers despite its history being "deleted". A nagging thought that I shouldn't be doing this submerges under a little thrill stirred in me by the search results. Porn sites fight for my attention with capital letters yelling out what they provide. I click Yahoo's video tab and start scrolling through, trying to gauge what each video might contain from its low-res thumbnail and very descriptive title, my free hand pulling my belt leather out its buckle.

62

'Don't you get bored?' Dad asks one afternoon he pops in for a sandwich and finds me drawing at the kitchen table.

'Yes.'

63

Thursday 29th November creeps up the calendar.

The night before, I get back from the gym, my arms sore and pumped, a vein running down each bicep. They're not smaller than before. No way.

'Scoot. Out.'

'The game's nearly over,' Jordan says, briefly taking his eyes off *Modern Warfare* to ask me for more time.

I take a fresh pair of boxers from my top drawer and go take a shower.

The gym's made me feel hungry, but the thought of tomorrow is stronger than a little hunger pang.

Mum takes me to college. We stop in the student car park over the road. It's a bright morning; I'm thankful she hasn't mentioned the Indian Summer.

Cutting between the throng of students piling in and out the front entrance, I'm petrified someone I know will see me with my mum. God, what if Sophia sees me? This is humiliating. We sit on the Bauhaus chairs beside Meeting Room 2. I pretend to look about, to sever any visible connection between Mum and me.

Boys in their sports hoodies and blinding trainers. Fighting and laughing. Shouting swearwords. They go through the lobby and out the set of automatic glass doors. How far have you come to be here? Doncaster? Gainsborough? Or are you from Scunthorpe? Are you a short walk from home? How are you comfortable, jumping about, swigging that Lucozade? Don't you think the things I do?

My trainers are muddy from walking through fields.

Mum sits still beside me.

First my personal tutor, Neil, emerges from the flock. A little buck-toothed and apologetic looking. He shakes hands with Mum and says hi to me. Pulls a chair up in front of us, as though we're going to have the meeting here in the crowded lobby, and asks if I'm alright.

'Think so, thanks.' I nod.

'What can you tell me, before we go in?'

'That I want to stay here.'

'That's what you want?'

His sincere stare and sloping eyebrows make me want to confide.

'I want to stay here. I know it doesn't seem like it, but I do. I'm not just skiving. It's not the same. I want to come but just can't.'

Before he can ask another question, the deputy head arrives.

A pistachio-green blazer and skirt. Foot fat that spills a little out of black kitten heels. Like how the head of a pint teeters just above the rim of the glass. A chirpy smile stretched over an undercooked dumpling. A cross between Margaret Thatcher and Professor Umbridge from the fifth *Harry Potter*.

I don't like her already.

'Bit brisk out today. At least it's brighter than yesterday. Shall we head in?' She gestures to Meeting Room 2. Shuts the door behind us and twirls the thing on the blinds until they're closed. Scooches round the table before leaning over it and offering her damp little hand. 'Nice to meet you. Nice to meet you. Oh!' She even shakes Neil's hand.

We sit opposite her. Neil repositions himself to our right; no doubt he doesn't want to seem on anyone's side.

You'd think the deputy would have important documents to tap straight and lay down, but no, a lone sheet of paper is placed under the table on her lap, out of sight.

'We're obviously having to chat about Chris's attendance, and it's become pretty dire.'

'I wasn't aware of it, my husband and I,' Mum says. 'We knew Chris was struggling to come into his classes and had missed one here and there, but we didn't know it was this bad. He's kept it secret. Now we're aware, I'm all for us sorting something out.'

'Absolutely,' murmurs Neil.

'What do you want to happen?' Deputy asks.

'Chris isn't himself,' Mum says. 'He went through secondary school without missing hardly a day, and at the start of his first year here—'

'His attendance still wasn't great,' Deputy butts in.

Mum didn't know that.

'It has certainly worsened, though. This isn't how he is. I'm not sure what the problem is, but it can't be ignored or treat like laziness. What *I'd* suggest would be cognitive behavioural therapy.'

'We can set up an appointment with our college nurse,' Deputy says.

I'm busy glancing side-on at Mum. What the hell's behavioural therapy? Where the hopeless trouble-causers in school used to go when they were kicked out of class? Will I be taught how to behave?

'Would that be Cathy Imogen? It would be a start,' Mum says.

Deputy faces me. 'What's stopping you attending class?'

'I don't know,' I say. 'I don't know.'

'And what's the outlook? What do you want to do in life?'

'I guess I want to be a writer.'

She laughs. 'The next J.K. Rowling? Isn't that a bit of a pipedream? Haven't you thought of something that would make a career? You know, we'd all like to be movie stars or famous footballers, but in the meantime we need to pay the bills.' She laughs again to Neil and Mum but they don't join in.

'Chris does writing because he enjoys it. Let's not trample on something positive he wants to do,' Mum says.

'Because, before we go down the road of help, we need to establish what we want here.'

'I want to stay at college.'

'I'm sure you do, but you're in A2 Level and you've missed eighty or ninety percent of your lessons. What expectation do you really have for the end of the year?'

'To pass. And do well. I might not be in lessons but I still work from home.'

'You can see my concern,' she says to Mum and Neil with a warm smile. 'We can have Chris see a counsellor and maybe that would help, but then what? How can he pull back his grades from the time he's lost? I hate to be realistic but the grades are what he's here for. Realistically, are you sure it's not better at this point to – you know – call it a day?'

The three adults look to me.

'No. I need to finish the A Levels.'

'I know you *want* to... We can get you started again next year.'

'Start all over again? What, from first year? No, I can't. I want to try to finish this year.'

'Is that really wise?'

'I mean I *will* finish the year. With this help you're talking about.'

She's expelling me. And trying to make it look like my idea.

The floor opens up under my chair, and I'm hanging onto the table edge.

'You can see my concern,' Deputy says.

Neil speaks up. 'With the college's support, I don't see why Chris can't at least give it his best for the rest of this year. We've got his best interests here, and he's interested in getting his grades. I'm happy to keep a closer eye on how he gets on.'

Deputy pushes her bottom lip one way, then the other.

'Let's see what happens, then. But at this point, his continuing here is conditional on him seeing someone to improve his attendance.'

Crossing the road on our way back to the car, even Mum says, 'She was a bitch.'

64

I'm in a corridor in college. Pacing about the corridor. Checking my insides with my mind.

It's a week since the meeting with Deputy. I have to see the head nurse in order to stay at college. A school fucking nurse. If I leave now, I'll be kicked out.

Mum's brought me in again: she's waiting in the car park over the road. But what if she leaves? What if she's already gone, and I'm abandoned here? And how fucking childish am I – driven here by Mummy to see the nurse – compared to the grown-up students swirling around me, their garish muddle of chatter like a waterfall of tin cans thrashing a cathedral floor.

The thick smells of college creep up my nose like cords.

Don't think about vomiting on this waxed lino, the distance to home, the people seeing you. If you think about it, it makes it worse, and if you make it worse, it might happen. Oh God.[20] It mustn't happen.

I'm in control. "The body follows the mind." That's right. That's what that guy said who could move things with his mind, and he started teaching others his meditation techniques. But then he got found out as a fraud who could make the smallest aperture with his lips and channel quick air through them to move objects. So why should I believe *him*?

I'm an island. "You're born alone, you damn sure die alone." That's what the guy on *Scrubs* said.

But I'm not alone, Emma's dangling off me. Not physically. She's in a lesson, somewhere. But I can feel her.

Pat my pocket. The pills are still there.

I try to swallow. I count everything I've eaten in the last few days. Which is almost nothing.

Picture yoghurt mixing with squeezed orange juice, curdling. Classic bars dipped in tea, their creamy middles melting. Gravy pouring from a boat. Picture being fit to burst with Sunday dinner, with the warmth of central heating working its way behind my eyes. The rubbery cheese that melts over a box of chips. Energy drink and chocolate bars. A Pot Noodle spilt across the road.

'Hi,' says the woman who's appeared. This must be Cathy Imogen.

'Hi,' I say, happy as anything.

She gestures into her office.

'Come in. Grab a seat. I'm just finishing a phone call but I saw you outside.'

Her desk faces a wall of notes thumbtacked into cork, posters about drugs and domestic abuse, reminders crowding a whiteboard; behind her, a handful of foamy staffroom chairs face a coffee table. I take the seat beside her desk, like being at a doctor's. The yellow colour schemes make me think of butter, clotted cream, sunshine. I

---

[20] Don't pray. You don't deserve to, listening to that blasphemous music. You spent your desperate prayer.

keep my eyes down. Green carpet. The doormat texture they use in schools. Like the one Simon Hislop puked up on when we were five. His vomit was pink; the lumps marinating in it looked like those polystyrene chunks that protect delicate packages. I could taste the smell.

Cathy picks up the phone and finishes a conversation about someone not wanting to go home, then puts the phone down. She turns her chair round to ask me what I'd bet she's already had the memo about.

'It's Chris, isn't it? I got a call off your tutor, Neil, outlining what's going on,' she says, 'and the deputy's sent through an email. So you've been missing a lot of classes, but it sounds like there's a bit more to it than that?'

'Yes.'

Trying to form a sentence threatens to strangle me to tears. It's like the episode of *The Simpsons* where the decrepit billionaire Mr. Burns is getting some medical test results, and it's both good and bad news: "You are the sickest man in the United States," the doctor says. "You have *everything*!" Mr. Burns has so many different, conflicting diseases, that none of them can actually get a hold and cause him any harm. The doctor demonstrates this with a number of small stuffed toys – or "oversized novelty germs" – which he tries to shove through a miniature "door to your body" all at once, getting them stuck in the frame.

There is so much to say that it's impossible to find the first word: the whole thing wants to cram through the door.

And at the same time, there's nothing at all to say.

'Why don't I let you fire away, then. What's the problem?' Cathy Imogen says.

Gathering words.

'I'm finding it really hard to come into college.' My voice is tiny. 'To do anything.' And that's all I manage. If I say another word I'll cry.

A microscopic answer inside her sprawling desert of a question, but it might keep me from being expelled.

Cathy nods. And when I don't add any more, she nods again.

'Okay. Does it make you nervous? Make you want to get out of here?'

I nod this time.

'That's okay. What's important is to know this isn't your fault, or anything to feel embarrassed about. We'll get in touch with the counsellor. You'll be able to talk about it to her and get to the bottom of it. Sound alright?'

Don't make me cry.

'Yeah.'

'I'd also email your tutors and explain the situation. You can copy me into the email in case they need it verifying. But I'm sure they'll understand. It's nothing that hasn't happened before. They may be able to work around your attendance.'

This is someone Mum knows. Has Mum mentioned her three boys to Cathy over the years? Spoke about us proudly, perhaps? Now Cathy gets to meet one. And look at him.

Jesus, Jane, you never mentioned that Chris was a little bitch, Cathy must think.

I write my mobile number down for her to pass on and that's that.

'Nice to meet you,' I say, now the urge to cry is ebbing. My voice still wobbles.

We exchange smiles and I shut the door.

The wind lifts my fringe up when the foyer doors open. I cross the road and find Mum's car. She puts away some work notes she was reading.

'She was nice. She's putting me in touch with a counsellor.'

'Good. That's a start then. Hey?'

'Yeah.'

She starts the car. 'Haven't you got any lessons to be in?'

Lessons! I'm starting to forget they exist. It's just gone eleven. I should be in Art in five minutes. The timing could be perfect.

'No, Thursday's always been an early day, remember.'

65

Part of me is proud. Being told to see a counsellor. It's mysterious. You know: maybe I'm a little unhinged. Maybe I have secrets.

But I instantly regret mentioning it.

'Why? Oh my god.' Ryan clutches his hair with a massive grin. We're in the Maggy May. 'Why're you seeing a counsellor? You've got to tell me.'

'It's honestly not that interesting,' I say. 'The deputy just said I have to go.'

'I can't believe it. You're like the new Zara Creswell.'

'Fuck off, am I!'

Zara Creswell was the crazy girl at school. Storming out of lessons, disappearing for weeks, even years, at a time. Never being punished, so it seemed. The teachers knew something. Then she'd return, appearing absolutely fine, before another outburst. We were quite terrified of her.

Ben comes through the automatic doors and spots our table.

'Chris has got to see a counsellor,' Ryan calls before Ben's even close enough to hear clearly.

In the next fortnight, she rings me.

Me, not my parents.

The counsellor's voice is brisk, precise. I like it.

She can squeeze in two meetings with me before Christmas. Two dates that I now watch out for. Two blips bobbing in the month of December. Times that I absolutely must go to college.

I pull the rolled newspaper from between the drawers and the wall. It's yellow now, like it's really old. Shit: I shouldn't touch this. It gathers more reasons, like rainclouds, not to go to college tomorrow. I open it out. A four-year-old toddler snatched during a family holiday. Tony Blair's reputation in shreds. Uncovering the tomb of King Herod.

'Look, look,' Jordan says behind me. He's playing *Modern Warfare*. 'Nine headshots away from blue tiger.'

'Fuck's sake,' I say. Which between us means, 'Impressive. Well done.'

'Who was on the phone?'

'No one.'

I lie on my bed and tell Emma about the counsellor over MSN.

I'm going to get better, I promise.

I'm here for you, she replies.

Hard frosts cover Barton. My feet don't sink into the grass or the mud. I break puddles with my heel. My hands stay up my coat sleeves, red and aching with cold. In the woods I squat on my heels and lean against a tree. Not long until the counselling. Things will get better. Just get through these days between here and then.

Then: the date of the final straw. I have to be in college, else I get kicked out.

A sour cramp of worry.

An **appointment**. A fixed slab of time with a professional. Just me and her. Unlike classes, where my absence might go unnoticed, not showing up to this would leave the counsellor sat there alone, getting progressively mad. She squeezed me into her schedule, only to be let down. Her time could've been better spent. I want the hour to arrive, if it will help me, but I'm scared shitless to go there. And these days between – I'm preciously clinging onto these days between, where not attending college won't guarantee expulsion. But I hate each one for the failing struggle it brings to go to regular lessons.

I revise every hiding place on the bus, the park between college and town centre, college itself. But can't stop picturing the sick spilling out of me. The putrid smell. The roaring disgust from everyone around me. Even the people on the top deck hear. Some peek down the stairs at the pale boy who doesn't know where to look. The pool of vomit trickles across the floor, between the plates of metal. It's a vision that re-arranges itself by the millisecond. Different angles. Different variations. In a classroom, in the Maggy May, with friends, beside Emma, in Sophia's sight, in Mum's car. Flicker, flicker, flicker. Diving out the counselling room. Finding a cup to be sick in. Finding a bathroom. Shit squirting out my arse in front of everyone. No control. Firing out both ends. A hot flush and light head reducing me to a delirious slump. Glimpses of misery. Re-arranged, repeated. Food, bacteria, clothing colour, air temperature.

66

'I'm finding it really hard to come in. I just – I don't know – can't do it. And it's not only college, it's everywhere.'

I say this to my folded hands between my knees. My throat constricts for a moment but nothing like last time. I'm not going to cry.

We're at the top of A-Block, in a tiny room overlooking the central square of college, where hundreds of students crisscross over the pavement to their lessons.

'By "can't do it", what do you mean?'

She's quite elderly. Early sixties? I don't know why but it surprises me. She's slim, droopy. Her cheeks have that slight Bulldog wobble when she moves her head or speaks. I wonder if, when she's bored, she can pull them closed like doors over her mouth.

'I – don't… It's hard to explain. I get really nervous.'

'A pressure to succeed? Like you'd feel before an exam?'

'No. Nervous at the thought of leaving the house. Getting on the bus. It's a really long bus trip to college, and I can hardly stand it. And when I'm here, it's like I'm stranded. I can't leave if I want to.'

'Why?'

'Because the bus only comes when college ends, at ten to four. And that's *so* long. Such a long time to be trapped here. And if I want to leave that badly, it's a proper hassle. I've got to walk into town or take a bus into town and then wait for another bus to take me home.'

'What is it about the bus that makes you nervous?'

Every answer takes time to come out. The words are solid.

'That it's enclosed. Once I'm on it, there's no getting off until you're there. Like, you *could* get off, but you'd be stuck somewhere remote between home and college. You're just trapped. Stuck in there. For however long the journey is.'

'Okay. And college is the same? You're trapped?'

'Yeah.'

'So are there times you're here but don't attend lessons?'

I sigh. 'Yeah.'

'Because that's worse?'

'Yeah. That's like… a cage within a cage. Within a cage. Classrooms are compact and full. And quiet. I wouldn't know how to just leave without stirring up attention. Everyone noticing me. Being weird and making a scene. And once I'm out the classroom, I'm still stuck in college, and if I make it out of college, I'm still stuck in Scunthorpe, or on a bus.'

One of her legs rests over the other. A black leather portfolio sits on her lap, bent open with a pad inside. She makes notes whilst I talk. Then taps her chin with her biro.

'Can you drive? Have you got a car?'

'No. Certainly wouldn't take the bus if I could.'

'Because that would mean you *could* leave whenever you needed to.'

'I know. Believe me. And I wish I had a car and could drive. It would make things easier. In fact this whole problem wouldn't exist. It would be ideal.'

'Well that's one thing to consider.'

'But lessons, the test, saving for a car. College will long-since be over before I get close to driving. I haven't got the money for lessons. And driving lessons are another thing I don't think I could do.'

'Because you're trapped in the car?'

'Yeah. With the instructor there. Maybe I could just drive us home if I wanted to. But I don't know.'

'A lot of people prefer the bus and trains to driving, because it's less to think about.'

'My mum says that. It's not how it works with me, though.'

She smiles.

'What about your parents then? Do you live with them?'

'Yeah.'

'How are things at home? Is there anything happening, or has anything happened, that might cause you to feel nervous like this?'

What a cliché, to ask about my parents.

'No, it's fine. I can't complain. I fall out with my parents over not being able to go places. They don't understand. They think I'm just not trying. You know, that I'm lazy or rebellious for the sake of it. That I spit their attempts to do nice stuff together in their faces. But there's nothing bad going on at home.'

'That's good. But you don't know what causes you to feel trapped in places?'

'No.' I think, then repeat, 'No. It's like I've always been this way.'

I should never have signed up for college, knowing I was like this. I should've known it would go this bad. I *did* know. Through Year Eleven I pictured it and felt scared, but assumed I'd cope when the time came. That I would have grown up by then. The line from 'Butterflies and Hurricanes' by Muse swung across my mind, "Your hard times are ahead", and for moments I felt ready.

'Well my key task here, what I'm employed to do, is get you into class. To find a way to make that manageable for you. *But.* There's no reason why we should ignore life outside of college. The two go hand in hand, don't they? If we can make you get on the bus and get into the classroom, who knows, it could help with everything else.'

It fascinates me how she takes a quick gasp before talking.

'Cool.'

She asks me more questions, then puts the pen down, laces her fingers round her highest knee and leans back until her arms are taut.

'So here's what I think. I think you've got a very active imagination. I think you take yourself too seriously.'

'Fair enough.'

'When you *do* make it through a day, or even to a lesson, do you reward yourself?'

'I haven't made it through a day since last year.'

'A lesson then.'

'No I don't reward myself.'

'Do you beat yourself up for not going?'

'Definitely. But not as much as when I'm letting someone I know down. My parents or my girlfriend. Then I just hate myself.'

'You shouldn't.'

'Why?'

'You're not doing anything wrong. The sooner you go easy on yourself, treat yourself well, the sooner you might recover.'

'Why reward myself for something that's *normal*? Not worth a reward, at least.'

'What's normal to others isn't normal for you. Everyone's definition of normal is different. If you were physically disabled and managed to stand up from your wheelchair and walk a hundred metres, wouldn't it be remarkable? I'm not suggesting you spend all your money on yourself every time you do something difficult. Anything small will do. Do you like chocolate?'

'Prefer sweets. Mints.'

'There you go. Buy yourself a little pack of sweets if you make it into a lesson. And if you make it through a full day, a big packet. You know, those Haribo ones. Deny yourself sweets unless you've achieved one of these things.'

'I get your point, but sweets are hardly enough to make me do stuff. When I'm worrying about whether I can make it onto the bus, I won't then think, *there's a bag of sweets at the end of the day waiting for me*, and magically jump on. What excites me way more, and I know it sounds sad, is being able to relax, knowing I've earned the right to relax. If that makes sense. I want to go home and make a tea and put the Xbox on feeling like I deserve to sit down. How I used to feel when I first started here, and would go home knackered at the end of every day.'

'That's not sad. Anyone worth their salt is proud of a full day's work. It's its own reward. I wouldn't know what I'd do if I didn't do this job, so I imagine it's hard to feel like your days are empty.'

'It is,' I say. She's hit a nail on the head.

'Then let's zero in on that. Throughout your day, keep checking in on that vision. That happy tiredness when the day is over. That's *your* tiredness, and you get to relax with it.'

It's a great thought.

'Shall we put the heater on? It's a bit cold.'

'Sure.'

She fiddles with the knob on the little radiator until a click resounds inside the metal. Runs a varicose hand over the grating. The smell of burnt dust percolates from inside.

'That's better. It gets cold in these upper rooms. I don't think they're connected to the mains. So, with what's called "positive reinforcement", you will start to associate the feeling of the bus, college, classes, with the pleasant feeling you get when you relax after a long day's work. It's a trick on the brain.'

'Won't my brain know it's a trick, since *I* know it's a trick, and I *am* my brain?'

'Let's test it out. So, what I want is for you to try coming into college, and giving yourself a reward for it. Then what we'll work on next time is a few relaxation techniques. Does that sound good?'

Try coming into college! Why didn't I think of that?

'Yep.'

The little knock at the front door.

Cold air follows Emma in. She kisses me and gives me a hug, and from the padding of her coat I breathe in the smell of the outside, the bus, college. She leans into the living room and chirps 'Hi' to my parents before following me upstairs. Unwraps her pink scarf, removes her coat.

'You alright? How did your thing go?'

'Yeah,' I say, leaning the pillow against the wall and lying on the bed. 'It was just her introducing herself and asking about me.'

Emma gets on, puts an arm and leg over me.

'What was her verdict?'

'She didn't have a verdict. She's suggested a thing to try, and she's going through relaxation things with me next time.'

'Is it anything like the print-offs I gave you? To do with anxiety?'

'Not sure.'

I never read that stuff. They went in the blue recycle box.

67

Granddad's oil paintings have been sold to hotels and museums; they line the walls of our extended family's homes, and they're all really good. Always historic. Boats, from the rowing kind to warships, in seas from stormy to glass-still; landscapes glowing in Constable sunlight; steam trains standing idle in busy old stations where the men wear top hats and the women hold up parasols; local chapels and churches before their pillage and collapse; Barton marketplace, Grimsby and Hull docks, hundreds of years ago, their industry bustling.

This little office is where he used to paint, and today we're gutting it. Me and Mum drag out every shelf, chair, the massive set of flat drawers for storing architect drawings, all his paints and brushes, the pots of turpentine I used to sniff as a child.

Being here makes me uncomfortable. Here in the presence of **old things**. The ancient food Grandma doesn't throw out. The old curtains and carpets releasing their spores. The woodlice and house spiders making their laps of the skirting boards. The green porcelain bathroom sinks no one's used in decades. The dried bars of soap with their dark crevices. The cupboard under the stairs that goes back and back, past the sweet-smelling blazers and that dead fox thing for hanging round your neck, past the tins and boxes and a thing you press to make dice jump around, to the tinkling toys we played with as fucking toddlers. The lights without shades and the lamps from India. Models of elephants rearing. The old writing desk with its compartmentalised ink pots, clam shells and human teeth. Foreign money and a block of graphite. The typewriters, the metal ship on the windowsill, fake plants stuck into those weird foam bricks that turn to sediment under the press of a finger.

Varnished bookcases line the walls of the main office. A small library of embossed golden titles on thick old spines. Filing cabinets full of Granddad's written work and research beside a wooden lectern. One armful at a time we take all the books downstairs and lay them in the lounge before Granddad, to choose which ones he wants to keep.

'I am loath to lose some of these,' he says sadly to himself. He does a few watery coughs into his balled hand. Reaches slowly down to the coffee table for his cup.

It's not just that one eye's gone and the other doesn't focus well even with his glasses: Granddad's interest in everything has dwindled. His painting has slowed to a halt; his reading and writing stopped. He doesn't have much to do with his mysterious fraternities anymore. He can't make the climb up and down his stairs to the offices unless it's really necessary. His energy is saved up for the nightly ascent to their bedroom. He used to complete the papers' crosswords every day, play alongside *Countdown* and record it on VCRs he organised into a majestic folding cupboard. He rode the stock markets. When I'd have a sick day in primary school I'd watch him read through the Teletext updates all day: fluorescent yellow and green lists on a black screen. Now he looks out the window and that's about it. Stares and stares. Up and down the road the cars go. Up and down the sun goes. On and off the streetlights shine.

We load the books into Mum's Fiesta. Granddad turns his chair round from the window to watch the pile shrink with each load we take to the charity shop.

I shut the boot, rub my fingers and thumb, rolling the thin film of dust that's accumulated in the clam of my hand into a cluster of little brown balls the size of salt crystals and flick them away.

We lug the shelves, cabinets and desk away from the office walls and throw dustsheets over them. I shake up a magnolia paint bucket and snap the lid up. This will be my bedroom. I note where the plug sockets are and wonder how I'll position my stuff. Tap the tired carpet with my toes. The floor sounds hollow; a stamp would shake every ornament in the house. What room's below this? The dining room. I can't shag Emma here – everyone will hear.

I text her the bad news.

Im sure we'll work around it ;) How long r u there for? Wanna see me tnight? xxxx she says.

I shut my phone and tip the paint into a tray.

With Granddad getting frail and Grandma struggling to maintain the place alone, we're prepping their house in case my family needs to move in at a moment's notice. We only live up the road, but Mum hates the thought of her dad having another fall and not being there.

Uncle Harvey still lives here, but he's in Cyprus at the minute with his new girlfriend – his cousin. Yes, we're all thinking the same thing. But Harvey's been alone for a long time.

Mum goes downstairs and I stare out the window for a while. The Humber Bridge lights arc over to Hessle. A train runs along the black far shore: a flatline across a heart monitor. It's Monday tomorrow. I can't go into college and reward myself. Not after being here. And then Tuesday I have to see my counsellor again, by which time the roots of infection will certainly have worked into me.

At home I check my inbox: my tutors have all replied to the emails I sent out explaining why I'm never there. Their responses are nice, even from my Literature tutor. And it's like dipping my toe into a sensation I can't explain.

68

The counsellor's name is Pru. In our next meeting she has me learn to take deep breaths. In through the nose, out through the mouth, holding in a full breath for a moment, holding out an empty breath for a moment. It feels nice.

'We can only really concentrate on one thing at a time, us humans. Concentrate on breathing, and you may still be nervous, but it's harder to think about it.'

'Okay.'

'So, have you managed to attend any lessons?'

'I went to English last week,' I say.

And even then, I got through a whole pack of Polos to keep the bile down. I sweated, fidgeted about on my seat, shaded in the margin of my notebook, touched the tablet bumps in my pocket, rolled a tear of paper between my finger and thumb. Studied the distance between the wall and the back of everyone's chairs who I would have to squeeze behind to reach the door whilst vomit tipped out my mouth.

One fucking lesson?! she must want to say.

'Did you reward yourself?'

'I didn't think attending one lesson in over a fortnight is reason enough to reward myself.'

'But it was hard and you managed it. That's worth an award. *Re*ward,' she corrects herself.

* * *

As the bus curls down the slope into Ferriby, I feel a sickness rising, so let's take deep breaths. Notice the quality of air. How it seems thicker passing through nostrils than it does the mouth. The smell of the bus coming in, the taste of my mouth going out. When the doors open, the cold air touches that delicate skin inside my nose; I can feel it go way up the tubes into my head, warming up, disappearing, then it leaves my mouth. Concentrate on it. The smells change between breaths: the dusty fabric of the seats, metal, an open bag of cheese and chive crisps across the aisle, the shampoo of the girl in front of me, the smell of Emma's house. Yes, Emma's beside me. She knows what I'm doing. She looks out the window, holding my hand. Her index finger strokes over my knuckle.

69

Middle of a December evening.

The gym windows are steamy. From the free weights area I watch how dark it is outside. Completely dark. Would my white skin betray where I am, even when it's night?

Ben recently joined. He was stick-thin, barely nine stone, like me before I started working out. But already I'm sure he's grown.

Instead of bicep curls and chest flyes, he sets up two stands, puts a couple of small discs either side of a long barbell and squats with the weight on his back.

'Jesus. How long do you manage in here?' Ben asks when we're in the sauna. He eyes the sand timer on the wall.

'Five minutes, usually. I've only managed the full ten once or twice. Eddy apparently had sex in one of these.'

'That's hard to believe.'

I let the back of my head gently hit the wooden wall. Sweat and water dribble down my neck, accumulate in my belly button. My arms are pumped.

'Where were you this morning?'

I fake a grin. 'Out past Spudders.'

'Spudders? Why?'

'To get pictures. There's this Media project we're doing where we make film posters.'

'They let you take the day off?'

'No. No, I'm just never in college anymore.'

'What's your attendance now?'

'Non-existent. It must be twenty percent. If that.'

'Aren't you worried? They'll probably throw you out.'

'Yeah.'

'Is it to do with the counselling? Why you're off, that is.'

'Sort of.' I stall.

'Is it something to do with why you won't sleep out?' he asks.

And that's the nerve. It makes my stomach drop.

'What?'

'How you never stay out anymore. I just wonder if it's something to do with that.'

'No. I don't get what you mean.'

'That's how it seems to me. How you've slowly stopped staying out, and now this. Is it to do with buildings? Like, houses? Whenever there's a house involved, you don't stay out. But when we used to sleep in tents or fields or the summerhouse, you did.'

'I stayed at yours, when was it, the end of Year Eleven? When Eeyore wouldn't have the window open.'

'But even then, you went at the crack of dawn. Absolute crack of dawn.'

Had I slept? It's hard to tell. I just lay there in the dark and reminded myself I had a house key if I needed to go home. It was raining and pitch dark when I walked up the roads back to my house, playing 'The Bright Ambassadors of Morning' through the cheap earphones I'd borrowed off Ben.

'All the times at Morgan's where you don't stay,' Ben says now. 'You've got to be the only one who hasn't slept there. And then Sutton. And Kenzie's party.'

'That was tents.'

'The barn one before that, though, too. So is it *open* places?'

'No.'

I sit forward, resting my wet elbows above my wet knees.

'Does everyone notice? Does everyone say things?' I ask.

'People wonder. There's always a reason. That's what people say. How there's always a reason you don't stop out.'

A big *thing* inches its way into the open. A big truth. I don't know how we suddenly got here. All the excuses I've woven, why I couldn't sleep out. Were they so obvious? I thought my secret was airtight.

'I don't think it's about where we are exactly, or whether we're indoors or in the open. I can't handle certain things. Situations where I can't *get away* if I need to. Like college, and stopping out places. Or going off to Sutton.'

Glancing up from the decking between my feet, I see a corner of Ben's mouth tuck into his cheek.

'Do you understand why?' he says.

'Not really. I get seriously stressed out and sick. That's all I know.'

Ben's hair slowly deflates under the steam and sweat.

70

The term is over, and college – let's be realistic – is a fucking shit show. I can't go in anymore. I can't fucking do it. I can't step onto that bus. I can barely do my sad laps around Barton, fooling no one. The fence of my enclosure is shrinking. Ferriby beach: that's too far, now. Down to Ben's house on a Friday night: it takes some doing. And in a sudden, terrifying projection, I see the rest of my life. College dissolving into nothing. My friends, James and Jordan going to uni whilst I stay here with my parents. And do what, get a job? If I can't show up to a lesson now, how could I do something so mandatory as turn up to a place I'm being *paid* to attend? And how many jobs, realistically, will never require me to go somewhere? It's not like working for Dad, who understands his son gets a bit funny at the idea of working anywhere but the yard. No. There are no lies I can spin in the real world, no wriggling out of the shit I'm afraid of. I'll lose my job. And every job to come. When I have kids, they'll want to be taken to the seaside, for a walk around a forest, out to a shopping centre. On holiday. If I feel Emma rattles along with me like chains, how will children feel? They'll *need* me. I can't leave them if things get too much. If I get ill, I'll be ill in front of them. Or be a father who can't leave the house. Who falls silent at the thought of doing anything fun. Who is unreliable. At the time they need me most, I'll get as far as the door and then mumble, 'I don't feel well'. I picture myself begging my parents to raise my children. My wife's disappointment. Would I *have* a wife? How could I keep one? How could I propose when even a trip to the restaurant would be too much to handle? How could I possibly stand still by the church altar, in front of hundreds, for her to make the painfully slow walk down the aisle? Will even Emma, with all her patience, grow utterly hateful of me? I bluff that she should move on. But soon, she really might. Shouldn't I have grown out of this now? A stupid thing I had as a child that's never gone away.

Is this **it**?

A deep nausea opens my eyes. But the images don't stop.

Every single scenario is detailed to a tee, each has preamble and context and far-reaching consequences. One scene inspires another, inspires another. Failure, misery, humiliation. Vomiting in front of people who used to look up to me, failing to manage basic responsibilities, trapped at home. No job, no money.

If I fail this year, it's the beginning of the end – a pit there's no clawing out of.

Two in the morning.

I pull my covers down, prop my pillow against the wall and sit up.

It's Christmas Eve.

The curtains glow faintly from the streetlights. It reminds me of being four years old, when I learned how to stop nightmares.

71

Dad's watching a shitty old film on the Freeview box, the sort reserved for Christmas Eve afternoon TV. Animatronic aliens tell a young boy they'd rather not stay on Earth because humans are illness-riddled. One of the aliens emphasizes the word *diarrhoea* like my Nanna does, and I feel infected by it.

A knock at the door – Sebastian's tall cloaked figure on the other side of the obscured glass.

'Answer it then,' Dad says.

'It's Eeyore.'

I hesitate. But he'll be able to see me, so I have to answer.

Sebastian gives me a card. I tell him I'm not well so shouldn't let him inside. He starts a conversation about music and Bitty, whose life Sebastian finds hilarious, but I manage to steer it to an end. He waves without his arm leaving his side and bobs away up the drive. I go back into the lounge.

'Are you doing the card run?' I ask Dad, opening Sebastian's to discover his signature drawing of a stick man inside a cube that he puts in every card.

Dad rolls a KitKat wrapper into a tight matchstick-sized roll. Turns his mouth down and shakes his head.

Part of me is sad – Christmas Eve card deliveries used to be me and Dad's tradition – but I'm also relieved. It would've been hard to go out visiting relatives, hence me saying, 'Are *you* doing the card run': I was poised to back out of it if this sickness gets any worse. Those dreams from last night are ringing in my ears.

Christmas cards become the topic of the hour. I find Mum and Dad talking in the kitchen. There's anger in the air.

'Read it,' Mum says, when I ask. She takes a little square Christmas card off the microwave and hands it over.

Jane and boys,
from Marie and Lowell.

Mum leans against the counter and her head shakes. Her sister and brother-in-law, Marie and Lowell Hobart, employed Dad for twenty-odd years to manage Bright-Spec, which in spring they secretly sold. When it came to light, Dad took it as his cue to leave too, but his exit ignited a backlash from the Hobarts that made no sense: they'd sold the company, and weren't anything to do with it anymore, so why should Dad be? Turns out, it was because Dad was unknowingly being sold too: he was part of the deal. That whole side of the extended family now say he's a traitor for leaving. The Hobarts are retired, loaded, playing the wounded victims.

Mum's stayed civil with her sister despite everything, but it seems a line's now been crossed.

'At least they sent something,' I try.

'What, this? Look at it, Christopher.'

She takes it from my hand and dangles it between a thumb and forefinger. There's a picture of a bauble on it. The card is bent in half, rather than folded with a clear seam.

'This *shitty* thing? With a few scrawled words. And no mention of your father. "Jane and boys"? They've sent it to show us they've excluded him. Like he's not in our family. It's disgusting.'

She Frisbees it and it slides under the microwave.

'Ah well.' Dad sighs.

'Don't you care?' I ask.

'Not really,' he says. 'I couldn't give a shit what they think of *me*. It's your mother I'm concerned about. I mean, that's her *sister*.

That's like James or Jordan sending you and your future family – well it's pathetic. Your auntie Marie and me had many a difference while we worked together but I've always considered her a woman of class. And now…' He gestures to where the card went and blows a dismissive raspberry.

'She'd write us a nice card every year. I would've got it if they didn't bother this year. That would've been, you know, whatever. But this is like a message. It's them saying that he's not only excluded from the wider family, he's not even part of *us* five. You, James, Jordan and I. Roping us as a family, against him.' Mum does more little head shakes. Her fury is so tautly reserved, it is pretty uncomfortable to be around.

In the night, the fear of falling behind keeps me awake again. I check the time: we've crossed into Christmas Day.

Dear God, let me not forget the real reason we celebrate Christmas Day. Help me not think it's all about getting presents.

A prayer that carries me to sleep.

Cross-legged on the living room carpet, I pull the wrapping paper apart to reveal an encyclopaedia-sized lime-green box.

'What on Earth's that?' Dad says from across the room.

'It's a program for making music on my computer. I can't believe it,' I finish to myself.

'Emma got you it?'

'Yeah.'

I turn it round in my hands. I'm overwhelmed. 'I can't believe it,' is all I can think to repeat, and send a bunch of thankful texts to Emma, wishing I'd let her join us here for Christmas Day like she asked.

The day after Boxing Day, Jordan lies on my bed whilst I play *Modern Warfare* and text Emma between matches. I don't know what courage comes over me, but I suggest going to visit her.

Jus for an hour. We're really busy with family christmas stuff xxxx, I lie.

Sure thats fine. Im all excited now! Teehee!xxxxxxxxxx

I clap my phone shut. Even though it's got at least a day's charge left, I plug it into the wall. What if I wind up needing to scrounge a sudden lift home and I've got no phone battery? I might be trapped between Emma's family members, where all I can do is send a secret text from my hip. I might burst out of her house, hide in a field, and have to describe my location to Dad.

It's ten past two. The sun will threaten to set in another hour; that's when I should head out. But if I head out *now* it'll still be dark by the time I've been there a while. And what if in *two* hours' time an illness overcomes me? I'll wish I'd gone sooner rather than later. Okay, then: maybe I should wait two hours and see how I feel, plus it'll be fully dark. No, because what if I'm ill *four* hours from now? It could strike at any time, let's face it. The shortest day is nearly a week behind me. I look out the window. Yes, it has to be now.

'I'll come for you in an hour, then,' Dad says when we pull up in the square outside Emma's.

'Yeah but can you be *here* an hour from now, not set off an hour from now? So, like, thirty-five past three?'

'Alright.'

On a stool in Emma's kitchen I glance again at the clock above the fridge, beside the crinkled painting of a misshapen frog her sister did as a child. Every minute is a strain to get through, like holding a press-up position. Her family's just finished eating. Plates waiting to be scraped litter the table; the counters and cooker are piled with pots, foil and chunks of food. They sit back and enjoy being full, whilst the thought of eating revolts me. I smile and laugh along to their banter. As usual, Emma's dad makes the odd lame joke and grins around the table. 'You'll have to get used to my dad's twisted sense of humour,' Emma giggles, leaning on me and snaking an arm under mine. I'm not sure what there is to get used to, but try to appreciate his talent to excavate primary school-level sexual innuendo from every fucking thing we say.

The family moves through to the lounge. Me and Emma talk and kiss in the kitchen. At half three, I start glancing at the window that overlooks the square. At thirty-three minutes past I open two fingers between the blinds, like they do in films.

'A watched pot never boils,' says Emma.

'Sorry. I don't want to keep my dad waiting. He seemed a bit impatient about ferrying me around,' I say.

Dad was perfectly happy.

'You could stay and I'll get Mum or Dad to take you back,' Emma says. 'I'm sure they'd be happy to if it means keeping you a little longer.'

'Ah, he's here. Too late.'

The Hummer's lights sweep across the terraces as Dad turns the car round and waits.

I poke my head into the lounge and say bye. Emma kisses me by the door and pretends not to let me leave. Pretends, but I still have to gently overpower her to escape.

At home I make a cup of Earl Grey tea like it's a ritual, thinking about what Pru said: after the hardship of Emma's, I *deserve* this cup of tea.

James and Bella watch *Pirates of the Caribbean: At World's End*. The characters sail The Black Pearl towards the edge of the sea, which pours over a horizon-wide waterfall into nothingness. When the sailors turn round to helmsman Captain Barbosa to demand whether he's sure about their suicidal direction, he shouts, "We're going in straight and true!"

The tea's bergamot steam dampens my nose when I take a sip.

Throughout the week, I stagger visits to Emma's: a day on, a day off. Each visit is barely an hour, so the clock says, but they are marathons to me. Emma asks why she can't see more of me. Doesn't she get how hard it is to manage even this?

Mum halts us in the square once again. I sit half out the car, twist the toes of my trainer on the ground, erasing the frost beneath my sole.

'So, can you be here *by* four?' The need to pull my leg back in, shut the door and go home sort of shouts all around me.

Mum's wearing leather driving gloves. 'That's barely half an hour.'

'Can you or not?'

'Yes,' she concedes. 'I'm meant to be at Grandma's but I might as well put it off until I've taken you back.'

Emma puts her hands up in a Y, standing on tiptoes, and hugs me. My cheek and nose rest in the soft skin where her neck slopes into her shoulder. It's her smell. The smallest wisp of comfort makes itself known.

In her room, she asks what I've been doing.

'James and Bella left this morning. I reckon that's all we'll see of him until after New Year's now. They're doing some party out in the sticks with their old school mates. Aw, man, I've been making *so* much music. I can import the crappy recordings I did on Audacity and make them so professional.'

'You've been doing more *Lord of the Rings* remixes.' She pulls the joking tell-me-the-truth face that normally annoys me, but I laugh this time.

'Maybe.'

Only hours ago, I shouted Jordan to my room, snapped my headphones on his head and watched him laugh himself beetroot red at my remix of "Looks like old Shelob's been having a bit of fun…".

'Taylor's tomorrow, then,' Emma says.

Taylor is a friend of our group we see once a year when he hosts the New Year's party, since his parents go away. He spends his waking hours playing Xbox. Waking hours that begin mid-afternoon and end in the early morning, as he doesn't work or go to college. He's rotund and softly built with a black gipsy moustache and half-closed eyes. He is the one who leaps to mind when I'm afraid of staying back a year at college, the one dwelling at the bottom of that pit I scramble at the mouth of.

'Yeah. Any time around half seven I reckon,' I say.

'Am I coming to yours first? I can get ready there and we'll go together.'

Why does she still ask this? Why make me repeat the same thing?

'I'll let you know.'

Mum's car is soon out the front. I unstick myself from Emma and the house, head down the path and over the square. The dark keeps me hidden. Freezing air keeps the nausea away. The Fiesta's rear lights catch the fumes lifting from its exhaust pipe.

'You're letting the cold in!' Mum cries over the gale of the heaters before my arse is even on the seat.

I clap the door shut.

The heaters are comforting: noisy, sleepy.

'Shall I just wait outside next time?' Mum watches me belt up, eyebrows high, one side of her jaw tucked into her neck.

We both laugh.

72

Midnight approaches at Taylor's. A bunch of people play Arrogance at the dining table. Ben and Holly disappear for a while, then a toilet flushes upstairs and Ben skids into the room, pumping a fist. Taylor has to drink a bottle of salad cream. His dog yaps and nips at our hands. Through the window it's already a hard frost; cigarette smoke looks thick and creamy in the side porch security light.

The TV gets switched over from *Guitar Hero* to the live count-down, and everyone starts finding their person to kiss, whilst the single ones make jokes that they have no one. Me and Emma hug in the middle of the lounge, watching the TV.

2008 isn't going to be a good year, I think, considering the state of the one we're leaving. But maybe 2009 will be alright.

Midnight arrives and we kiss.

Part 2

1

The hours before term begins are below triple figures.

Our living room TV's perpetually left on. I go to switch it off again only to find it's showing a news headline about a sickness bug sweeping the country. Now I'm perched on the arm of the chair, thinking, is this the last nail in the coffin? The deal's sealed: I can never go back to college.

Turn it off before the report starts.

No, I need to know.

It'll make it worse to know.

Not as much as not knowing.

The presenter passes the headline on to the correspondent, to open it into the full story. She's stood on a shiny studio floor. She says the words *sickness and diarrhoea*. Is she *emphasizing* them? And before there's time for the news to sink in, they move on to the next fucking story.

How can they report this without causing panic? And tell us so little?

Either tell us nothing or tell us everything!

Is the virus in the air? On our skin? On the objects we touch?

Yes, yes, and yes, of course. I know this.

2

I wake up tired. It's been another night staring at the door, seeing the future.

Dad's in the living room, which is odd. He's usually at work well before I wake up. He'll be in the office as early as four to get a head-start on the workload.

'Thought I'd actually go in for eight this morning. For a change,' he explains. 'Sod it.'

Whenever he's in that seat, he picks his nose. There's no exception. Every fucking time. A big old finger roots for bogies, pushing out the side of his nose, like no one can see. Whatever gloopy scab he finds is then rolled between thumb and finger for a minute or two. Sometimes he's got both hands rolling bogies at once, like he's tuning in an invisible ham radio. Once the specimen is a dry ball, he flicks it away. It might be sticky, taking two or three flicks to clear his thumb.

I never sit in that seat. Nor on the right-hand side of the sofa, which is potentially in range of his flicking trajectory. Nor do I touch the cushions he keeps on his lap. I try to turn myself so the picking ritual is out of sight, especially when I eat, but you can't see the TV screen without the digging and the rolling in your peripheries. And it's not like I can turn and face the wall: questions will be asked. I don't confront him because I'm embarrassed to acknowledge I'm witnessing something personal. Unlike Dad, apparently. Many times I've come in and been relieved to see he's not picking his nose, but then, as though my presence has reminded him of a job he needs to do, up goes the finger.

'Where's your breakfast?' he asks today.

'Had it already,' I lie.

The bus pulls into my stop in an hour. That's time enough to excite my stomach if what I eat is off. And a bus ride whilst sick is an unbearable thought. Then again, so is being sick at its destination.

So when *can* I eat?

Let's be generous and say food poisoning and/or a bad reaction to food manifests itself in three hours. Shall I eat at about two o'clock, then? That way, if I'm poorly, it'll be at about five and I'll be at home by then. Unless the bus is late or breaks down. Okay, I won't eat until I'm home tonight. I'm alright to eat then, surely? Sure. Unless the effects of tonight's food spill into tomorrow morning.

After how many hours can I say with certainty that the food I eat has not made me ill?

Horrible Science books taught me that food is fully digested in six hours. Let's say I'm safe by then. Six hours. But if the food's fully digested, will I have to take a shit at college?

Okay, I'll remember not to eat until it's less than six hours before I'm home. That's eleven in the morning I can have breakfast, if I'm *sure* it won't upset or poison my insides. Let's say poisoning's window of revealing itself is between three and six hours, and take it from there.

But don't people have dinner in the evening and then feel poorly in the morning? That's, like, eight to twelve hours. Don't people go *well* into the next day, still saying, 'Man that curry last night isn't agreeing with me'?

In fact, was it Bethany who, during a conversation about the pink centre of a Dixie Chicken breast she once bit into, said food poisoning can suddenly kick in after six months? She could be right. Am I only safe six months after the food in question enters my mouth? Must I remember everything I've eaten in the last six months? If I eat something I'm suspicious of, should I play it safe and not leave the house for six months? If I'm sick after three months, does that mean the poisoning is over, or should I stay indoors for the remaining three months of the six-month period? Being sick doesn't *mean* it's food's fault, after all. It could've been a virus, and the poisoning is yet to come.

A virus. The virus is still around. How long before it's gone? A few weeks? How much warning does it give before you explode from mouth and arse?

'It just came over me out of nowhere!'

Dad goes for his morning shit and I carry on watching the ancient fishing programme he's got on. I lift my glass of water off the carpet and lean it on my mouth enough for the drink's surface to wet my top lip. Not quite a full sip. Tea or coffee are out of the question. Neither have caused an upset stomach in my life, aside from that scare on the way home last year, but today might be the first day. My eyes flit between the digital clock on the VCR and the wooden one on the mantelpiece.

Through the wall, the toilet flushes and the bathroom door opens. Surely that wasn't enough time for him to wash his hands. Does he wash before flushing the chain? I hear his shoes on the kitchen floor. The fridge opening. Mum talks to him.

I go upstairs and style my hair. Normally I do this knowing no one will see me today. But that's got to end.

Half seven. Jesus.

Check my reflection again.

Check my bag for everything I need.

Check the side pockets for the tablets.

Check my stomach. It's hollow, a vacuum pulling in my belly button. I touch the bone plateau where my ribs end and the soft slope down to my belt begins. Go through to my parents' room and check Mum's alarm clock. It's time.

The closing half of 'Piggy' by Nine Inch Nails echoes in my head. "Nothing can stop me now, 'cause I don't care anymore," Trent Reznor chants. Again and again. A chorus, a mantra, a conviction.

"Nothing can stop me."

This is the very edge of the descent down to nothingness. I *must* get through a day.

'You're not going, then. It's back to the routine,' Dad says when I'm in the kitchen grabbing my shoes.

'Why are you saying that?'

'Isn't your bus at ten to?' He nods to the oven clock.

I jam my feet into my trainers, hopping down the hallway, and clap the front door behind me. My legs are weak and notice the tiny incline on our brickwork drive. I run to the end of the street and spot a few people still at the bus stop. I cross the road and ask the sixty-odd year-old woman amongst the students if the Scunthorpe bus has come yet.

'No. It's late,' she says. 'As always.'

'Lucky for me.' I smile.[1]

'I'm off to my daughter's. My husband can't drive so I'm having to take bus. She works, you see. And someone's got to take care of little one while she does.'

I only asked if the bus has come.

'Good job she's got you.'

---

[1] Nothing can stop me now, 'cause I don't care anymore. Nothing can stop me now, 'cause I don't care. Nothing can stop me now, 'cause I don't care anymore.

'I know! Can't rely on the dad. No, I shouldn't say that. He's at work, too.' The old lady laughs. 'Is it college you're off to? Of course it is.'

'Yeah, Leggott.'

'You go for it. Jesus, I wish I'd gone to college.'

She adjusts the golden handbag over her shoulder and an object drops out.

'Damn it.' She squats down.

'I'll get it.' But as my fingers stretch down to the tarmac I see it's a panty liner, and I falter.

'I'm sure it'll be here in a minute,' she says, standing back up, looking down the road to where the bus comes from, tucking the pad into her bag.

Emma looks surprised to see me when I get on the bus.

Three times on the journey in, my skin flushes, my stomach squeezes, like I'm about to vomit.

"We're going in straight and true!" Captain Barbosa shouts in my head, above the gales of a storm at sea.

I let the door to the Media Studies room close behind me. I smell the floor wax and heaters, the dust, the humans.

Third floor. Two in the afternoon.

It's happening: an afternoon Media Studies lesson.

There's a small cluster of desks pushed together and fifteen students sat round it. I find a seat, pull my writing pad out.

The conifers, there out the window, on the far side of the sports field: I'd almost forgotten about them.

'I'm milk sick. You know when you get milk sick? Had a whole bottle between Philosophy and here,' a girl with marshmallow cheeks says.

'You have the stomach of woman,' her friend declares. He runs his palms forward and backwards over the table as far as he can reach, sits back, sits forward, chewing gum behind a big smile and wide eyes. Well shit, it's the boy who threw that diabolo above the building and caught it, back when I first started college.

By the time our teacher comes in, I've already drawn a few inches up the margin of my notepad. This is the first time I've met him, the first time I've attended this class that began in September.

I munch Polos and towards the end of the two-hour lesson take today's fourth dose of paracetamol to see me through the journey home. The sun goes down. The dark conifers become harder to see against the blushing sky. Glover Road's streetlights come on, and I wonder if our bus is down there waiting for me yet.

When I close my notepad, I notice I've written "This is" on its cover, and wonder when I wrote that, or what it meant.

'Hellooo, Chris,' the teacher says once everyone's left, putting on a deep, gloomy voice.

'Hey,' I laugh.

'I got your email. Did you manage alright today?'

It's fucking Baltic on Glover Road. Emma goes 'Ooooh!' and pinches her eyebrows at me. She stamps her heels on the tarmac, unzips my jacket and threads her arms under it, around my back. I put my chin on her head.

It's as good as dark, but I see a peach sky behind those brick chimneys, beneath the black clouds.

'Love you,' says Emma.

'You too.'

She wears her pink scarf. Her straight hair falls over it.

I bow my head so it's next to hers, my nose nuzzled in the scarf, and catch myself enjoying her smell that rests in its warmth. I forget about the strip of peach sky.

The bus arrives twenty minutes late.

Sophia and her friends run a few steps up and down the kerb, guessing where it'll stop, to make sure they are first on. The doors *pisssh* open and they run straight up to their spot at the front of the top floor with pretend desperation. They're joking, but also not, I reckon.

Emma finds us a seat. She sits by the window, folders laid on her lap. I put my knees up. Sebastian slinks on and sits in front of us.

Before we're out of Scunthorpe, our bus dragging itself up the winding hill to the mental home and Roxby, it's black outside. Emma leans on me and I pick up an end of her pink scarf. Last year, when we'd journey home together every night, we would make plaits out of my scarf's tassels.

'Nothing to plait with this one,' she says.

I pinch one of the tiny wool bobbles from the scarf's fuzzy knit. Roll it between my finger and thumb until it's condensed into a tighter sphere. I place it in Sebastian's hood. Emma nudges me and I laugh. Pinch another bobble and do it again. Pinch another and put it in Emma's hands. 'Nooo,' she says in her high pitch, barely audible above the bus's protesting engine. Gently take her wrist and guide her hand forward and then shake it. I can feel Emma laughing. She drops the bobble into the hood.

By the time we're through Winterton, Sebastian's black coat appears to have measles.

3

My personal tutor Neil, who helped persuade Umbridge/Thatcher from kicking me out of college, catches my eye and nods. I hang behind after Tutorial and he comes to sit on my desk. He's got buck teeth inside a kind smile; rectangular glasses nip his egg-shaped head. 'Good to see you here. For the first time, is it?'

'Almost.' I nod.

'How many lessons have you managed?'

'All of them.'

'*Really*? What's changed? Your counselling?'

'Not sure. Maybe. I can't really think why.'[2]

'When are you next seeing her?'

'Next period, actually.'

'Oh, smashing. Great. So, did you need to chat about anything?'

---

[2] Nothing can stop me now, 'cause I don't care anymore. Nothing can stop me.

'Yeah. I know how late I am for this, but I want to apply for uni.'

'It is late in the day. Not *too* late. The deadline's next week.'

'I didn't think I would go. But – it was over Christmas. You know, I decided. I've got to go. I've got to get in.'

'First job's to round up references, then. You'll be wanting everyone who taught you last year as well as this year. Do you have a university list in mind?'

'Think so,' I say, having done a mad search last night for universities that teach Creative Writing. 'Every teacher probably hates me for chasing after my attendance all year.'

'I'm sure they don't.' Neil shakes his head and a fucking ponytail whips out from behind his bald dome.

Pru stokes up the radiator in our tiny counselling room.

'What's changed? Have you kept up with the relaxation exercises?'

'Yeah, but I honestly don't know why I've been coming in.'[3]

It must be a curveball, because Pru doesn't have much to offer for the next forty-five minutes. It's like she's padding the time out. She leans me back to go through a relaxation technique, she reminds me what to do when I get nervous, and that's that. I watch the college square below us darken, and its spherical white lights come on.

Emma finished early today. She asked if I wanted her to wait around until the end of the day, and I said something like, 'No, don't do that for me.'

Glad to be alone, I walk to Glover Road. The bus is twenty minutes late again. Are the drivers on strike? It's freezing enough to make me grateful when it rumbles to a stop and we pile aboard. I put my earphones in and select *Sound of Silver* by LCD Soundsystem, which James got me for Christmas.

Through the grimy windows, through a nick in the cloud, I spot yellow sky[4] before it falls completely dark. I look into the dark and soak it up, thankful for every minute of invisibility it offers. In a few

---

[3] We're going in straight and true!

[4] The colour of whisked egg, which reminds me of egg yolk, drooling or half-set, which makes me uneasy.

months, the sun will be high at this time of day. On the flat fields of the Ancholme Valley, the spot-lit cement works come into view – silos and conveyor belts floating in the dark. The *nearly home* feeling melts over me, like reclining, like the sudden absence of pain.

Mum arrives home at eight, after another twelve-hour day. She turns the hob on. 'Going to dolly-up last night's pork into something,' she says, clopping about in her shoes.

When we're eating, Dad asks, 'What do you reckon to Devon this summer? Your mother and I are thinking Finlake again, rather than a repeat of that *Scheißen Haus* down in Hale. A week in Devon. And *then* up to Surrey for another week, in Tilford. Near Bourne Woods, again. What do you say? I know it's not Florida.'

'Ah, right,' I say.

Finlake's a resort of cabins on the side of a wooded hill on Dartmoor. We went there when I was little. A steaming pile of memories land on me: endless traffic jams on the drive down, getting to know the cars that inch along either side of us, long walks and days out, miles from the hut. Tilford's a little village in Surrey; we stayed there in a hut a few years ago. I took Ben's dad's laptop to watch episodes of *Friends* on DVD and write my book. It's a train ride away from London, a trip I already know my parents will want to take again.

'Cool,' says Jordan.

'"Cool" as in "yes"?'

'Definitely.'

'Chris?'

Even when being friendly, him saying my name is still a little stab.

'Sure.' I keep my eyes down on my gravy and pork.

Upstairs, Jordan plays *Call of Duty* and I read through the mark scheme of a Media assignment.

Devon, then Surrey. A fucking double holiday. At some point, I'll have to break it to my parents that I can't go. It's too much, too far. If they could only be convinced to go without me.

But with the house free, Emma would want to stay the night. Or the *fort*night.

I could keep it secret, and be utterly alone.

'Have you got red tiger on everything?' I say to Jordan, peering over the top of my laptop to see the TV screen, where his soldier pop-shots another player in the head with a red and black-camoed assault rifle.

'Mm hm.' And as though it accompanies his answer, Jordan inflates his cheeks to stretching point and makes his nose retract into them without turning from the screen.

'How the hell are you doing that?' I shout, and his cheeks burst as he starts laughing.

4

A hint of light finds the naked trees I step between, careful down the frost-sharpened mud path. Scorched glass shards pop under my foot in the "turbos" clearing on the fringe of Tree Field. I sit on a low trunk that's grown horizontally. It's Friday morning, and I was too sick to catch the bus. But I've been to four out of five days this week. That's good, surely. I can give myself this day off. A reward.

This is a failure, not a reward.

A step closer to the bottomless pit's brink.

Was I *really* unable to make it into college today?

Now there's a whole weekend before I can try again. And time off is space to think and worry, to return to how I was.

As Dad said the other day, 'It's back to the routine.'

The dog walkers will come this way soon. I mustn't see them.

At home, I sit at the piano and begin to loop around 'The Entertainer', but stop after a few seconds. I walk through the living room and detest the thought of turning the TV on. I shouldn't be here.

An hour later I feel the aching urge to watch porn and have a wank, but I don't. Something isn't right about it.

In the evening, Dad drops me off at Emma's.

'You sure you don't want any?' her mum asks, a spatula of chips in her hand.

'No, thanks. I've already had dinner before I came.'

Dried old crumbs litter the kitchen table, as though hoping to attract birds. I take a seat and look at the big tub of melted butter Emma's dad scoops onto his bread roll. He then dips the roll in ketchup and thumbs a few chips inside. It's so hot here. The smell of food, the consumption: it's pressing down on my chest. A threat of panic buzzes in my limbs, my guts, my hair follicles. I picture jumping up and running out the door into the dark.

Emma pushes away from the table and blows out with her cheeks puffed.

'May I be excused? Thanks very much for tea. Shall we go through, Chris?'

'She always gets out of washing when Chris is here,' Emma's older sister Miranda says.

'Don't be a mardy cow,' her dad says, then starts cackling at Miranda's scowl until Miranda laughs too.

Emma's mum leans backward to see me from behind an open cupboard door. 'Do you want a cuppa?'

'Not just now, thanks.'

One hour thirty-five minutes since arriving, my phone vibrates. I go outside where The Hummer's waiting inside its own slow-turning choke fumes.

'We're off to see James tomorrow, your mum and I. Fancy the ride out?' Dad says as we creep down Emma's street.

A little girl pushes an empty doll's pram. She stops to watch us turn out.

'Don't think so. I should do work,' I say, knowing I won't.

'You've got to come *some*time, mate. Eh? James would be over the moon.'

'I know.'

We're halfway through his first year and I've never seen James's "digs". I miss him, but can't go to Nottingham. Two and a half hours away. I only see him when he comes home for a night, every couple of months. He lives in student halls, and I love hearing about the crazy parties they go to that start in a half-wrecked flat living room, pre-drinking any no frills spirits they can afford, then spilling out into the streets, hopping from club to club until morning; the pranks James and his friends on the corridor pull on each other; the Russians who for a few hours a night sit on top of the main porch drinking vodka and always say, 'Hail, Westy,' whenever James arrives. Real stories. He's loaded with them whenever he comes home. James wants me to go stay over with him and join in. And I want to. I want stories to tell. Every anecdote I tell is about a friend, a brother, or even someone my friend knows, someone my brother knows. What have I got to say? 'The other day, I walked around Barton, played piano, played Xbox.'

What does Sophia get up to?

We pass the bollard lighting up Gordon Brown's stencilled face, onto the main drag home.

5

'We'll have to chop them trees back again when spring comes. Me and Jordan. Whack some of those nettles down with sticks like we used to. They've overgrown since last year.'

At the word "sticks", Granddad notices me here on the sofa arm in his living room. He snaps round from the window to face me so quick, looking so shocked, my last few words wobble with laughter.

'Ah, yes,' he says. He gently nips his bottom lip and relaxes deeper into his chair again, gazing out the front window. 'Very good.'

It's strange. By now he should be telling me where the manpower to build Lincoln Cathedral was amassed.

What's he looking at?

Perhaps the paper birch on his front lawn, with its stout white trunk and wet black branches fountaining out the top, its twigs tickling the top of Mum's Fiesta, parked beneath it. Ferriby Road, and the cars zipping up and down. The semi-detached houses on the other side of the road.

Mum steps in wearing blue marigolds – the sort she'd never buy for herself. In one hand's a scourer. She wipes her brow with the back of her forearm. Spots me and nods, then goes back to carry on cleaning.

The carpets downstairs are flattened to the concrete; some have those dark Indian patterns from the 60s, others are a custard colour, stained here and there with the spills of grandkids' ham-fisted eating. The walls are all white, the decorations scarce. Big empty rooms that amplify small sounds. From hints and eavesdropping over the years, I gather Grandma and Granddad are pretty rich. But they were affronted by Mum's tactful suggestion of a few new carpets and a fresh layer of paint.

I drag more boxes into the spare bedroom, careful of the pins on the carpet. Ornaments crowd an ancient dressing table; drawers lined with red felt hold ivory-handled hairbrushes and forgotten tubs of Vaseline. There's a stale bed with salmon sheets, a secret cupboard and a smell I can't place. Next door is Uncle Harvey's room.

'What are these?' I ask, when my pulling bends the wall of a box enough to peek inside.

'More of Granddad's essays,' Mum says. 'Notebooks, a load of diaries from sometime back whenever. Don't start rooting, I've just finished packing them.'

But I open a small navy-blue leather journal that looks different to the sort I know Granddad to write in, where most days are now blank.

'Jesus, Mum. Nineteen thirty-two.'

Old paper smell emanates from within. It makes me imagine minute particles of dust and fibres of pressed wood floating up my nose, settling on the moisture of my lips.[5] The skin that shed into the pages and rotted. I want to read his fine pencil italics – I glimpse Granddad travelling alone, learning as an occupation, a mobility I can hardly associate with the person he is now – but I also want to return it to where it can't be touched, and wash my hands. But

---

[5] I must remember not to lick them until I next have a shower or wash my face.

remember: the old green porcelain sinks of my grandparents' many bathrooms. The bars of soap with dark cracks.

Ryan, Ben and Boris come up to my place later. Boris plays *Call of Duty* whilst me and Ben talk. Ryan has his feet up with my laptop rested on his legs, keeping quiet, occasionally dipping the end of his finger up his nose.

'Look at Ryan, pulling his bottom lip,' Ben says.

Ryan holds up his middle finger without looking up from the laptop.

Ben prowls behind Ryan to see the screen.

'What're you – he's got porn on! What the fuck? What the *fuck* is—' he hangs his head, a hand on Ryan's shoulder to stop himself keeling with laughter, and manages to take a breath '—"Cum on toast"?'

Ryan tips his hands outwards. 'I just found it.'

Ben sits against the drawers and wipes his eyes. His voice goes up an octave: 'C – Cum on fucking toast!'

Boris pauses the game. 'Let's have a look.'

Ryan's a shade redder but he doesn't budge.

I laugh along without going to see the video. I make a mental note to clear my internet history later, not because of someone thinking I've been watching that video, but because the laptop seems tainted. It's as though an act that feels *wrong* has been done with it and if I don't erase the evidence soon, the blame will be mine, too. It could mean I become sick.

6

The smell of wet clay, paints, white spirit. A girl a few rows behind me uses a hairdryer to harden a layer of acrylic, and my eyelids become heavy.

I snip a rectangle of canvas from the roll, give it a base coat, dry it off whilst trying to picture the vantage point I had just before our bus snaked down the hill into Scunthorpe this morning. I could see the lights of the whole town; everywhere else was pitch black. I paint a bright circle, then slowly creep the blackness in around it, snuffing the light, shaping it into a version of that view.

After Art, me and Emma walk up to Spar together and I get a pack of Polos. She's meant to have an early day today but announces she'll stay and wait, in case I'm free to see her after college. No pressure, then. If she comes, at least that might keep her from asking again until the weekend. Half the Polos are chomped by the time we're back in the Maggy May.

We find the table where a few of our friends are sat. Anyone seeing Ben for the first time today gasps and laughs, patting his crew cut where the massive afro bobbed about only yesterday. It shows off how much weight he's packed on; since he started lifting, he's had to replace all his old clothes, because nothing but his socks still fit.

'I always do this thing with mints,' I say to Emma, 'where I flip them like this between my top and bottom teeth. Like, pushing it with my tongue. It gets going proper quick, flipping like this, and you can eat the mint quicker without crunching it. See? Watch.'

Emma laughs.

'It just looks like you're chewing it.'

'No, see. One piece. Again, watch.'

'Can I have one?'

She takes one out the packet and sits under my arm. It takes me a minute to notice that every time I face away to talk to someone else, she pokes the mint out between her lips, like sticking out a little white tongue, then sucks it in when I look down and see her. I wait until she thinks I'm not looking and lunge for the mint she's sticking out again. Emma sups it out of reach and sits up, laughing and half-choking. She turns round with a tight-lipped smile and sticks the mint out at me again.

We've turned the wrong way. This isn't the way to Barton. I look about the bus. Hasn't anyone noticed? Is it a shortcut? Is the driver getting us lost?

'We're off the wrong way,' I say after a few minutes.

'Are we?' Emma asks. 'It's dark, how can you tell?'

We cross over a junction, head past the posh windmill restaurant, turning round a tight bend and through some gates, into a bus depot, to a halt.

'Someone's been sick upstairs,' people start to say.

'A girl's been sick upstairs.'

Rows of buses extend either side of us, as though we're parked between two mirrors.

Is it true? Why was she sick? An infection, a virus?

Will it trickle through the ceiling onto our laps, our scalps, like the rain does?

Don't get carried away.

Keep your head down! If you look up, it might drip into your mouth.

The driver opens the doors and hops down into the night, comes back and sparks up a fag, leans against his bus and watches in the direction he walked from. A man arrives out of the dark with a bucket, mop, tray of cleaning products. There's a slow-building '*Whaaay!*' as he steps aboard, that reaches its loudest as he climbs the stairs and the top deck sees him. 'Wish I had your job, mate,' someone calls.

We're moving again. I make sure to breathe through my nose[6], but keep the breaths shallow.[7] We trundle between the high walls of the cinema and car park, and I feel a burning in my stomach. Should I stop eating so many Polos?

Emma gets off at my stop. She eats bolognese with us. We cuddle in my room, I lick her out, I say there's work I should be doing.

That was three hours she was here, I think, once Emma's left. A whole day of college *and* three hours with Emma. What a span of, what's the word, stress-time, danger, being offshore. Like all my

---

[6] Breathing through the nose is far better at stopping airborne germs from entering your body than breathing through your mouth. Ben once said, 'If less people breathed through their mouth, colds wouldn't spread half as easily.'

[7] Dreading the smell of vomit. To smell is to receive molecules of a substance through the nose. So if I smell the sick from upstairs, it means I'm taking a fraction of it in. Vomit molecules. From their ill body to mine.

muscles were tensed the whole time, and it's not until this moment that I can let them relax. I can stop thinking about escape routes and terrible situations. It's safe to stand down.

I play Xbox for a while, feeling like it's truly earned. But what about the girl's vomit on the bus: was it an airborne illness that may have floated down the stairs to me? The sickness bug they reported on the news?

7

'I missed Friday, last week. The day after we spoke, in fact.'
'Why?' Pru asks.

'Back to my old ways,' I say, and then wish I hadn't, in case that's actually true. 'I'd been thinking about college into the night. And it became so, like, daunting. But I'm not sure about the main reason. I saw the bus stop and couldn't get on. I kept walking.'

She tilts her head to the side and nods.

'You look disappointed in yourself.'

'Maybe.'

'But what's that going to do to help?'

'I don't know. Might remember how disappointed I felt on Friday and that might stop me missing a day next time I'm really nervous.'

'Maybe, but you said how terribly disappointed your family were with your attendance, and how upsetting that was. Yet it wasn't enough to make you come to college, was it?'

'No.'

'No. There's being *tough*, resolving to do better next time, and then there's beating yourself up. Don't do the second one. You relapsed. After an otherwise brilliant week. A relapse doesn't mean you're back to square one. A relapse is included in the path to victory. You managed four days and fell short on one. Isn't that good?'

The radiator ticks and dings as it heats up.

'I guess.'

'And here we are. Tuesday, on week two of spring term.'

Spring? Don't mention spring.

'My family's also announced we're going on holiday this summer.'

'Good?'

'Not really. I can't – how can I do that? It's down in Devon. I'm barely managing to come twenty-one miles to Scunthorpe.'

'How would your family react if you didn't go?'

'I don't even know. They'd probably refuse to go themselves.'

That image of me and Emma in a free house swirls together with the memory of the Spurn Point day.

8

We're at our Maggy May table.

My bag's leant against my chair leg. I glance down at it when Ant shuffles in his chair. Let my arm hang down and hold one of the straps. Check the zips are fully closed.

'Have you seen the new Leggott Porn?' Cartwright says.

A few of us say yes. I say no.

There was a Leggott Porn last year, circulating around anyone with a Bluetooth phone. It found its way onto the internet too, I reckon. Apparently the girl in it was in Ryan's biology class. Never saw it myself.

'It's going round, man.'

Ryan and Ben start laughing. They lean into each other, tap each other with the back of their knuckles, like they do.

'What?' I ask.

'The video,' Ben says. 'The girl goes, "Do me from behind," and the guy goes, "Up your arse?" and she goes, "…No." Then his cock starts going down and you hear him whisper, "Help me!"'

Everyone laughs.

'You see blood on his thumb, though.'

'Yeah, I saw that,' Cartwright winces.

'I'm missing out,' I say.

I never want to see it. It doesn't seem right that I see it.

It's nearly ten past two. Students on other tables start to get up, and a wave of those now on a free period file in through the doors.

Most people hang their bags over the back of their chairs in here, but that way, someone might open it whilst your back's turned. People do it for fun, and even take stuff out. And *no one* can discover the tablets in mine. It's the same with my pocket. Should my knees be too high whilst sitting, it could tilt my small pocket enough to tip the pills out. I might be left in a situation where I direly need them, only to discover they escaped my pocket earlier. Or, almost as terrifyingly, I could be sat here in the Maggy May with friends and they tip out, revealing to the world that I keep anti-diarrhoea tablets in my pocket. I imagine scrambling to the floor to grab them, but everyone's already seen the labels.

I touch my pocket again, feeling for the little bumps, pick my bag up and head over the courtyard, past the pond and the old smoking shelter.

In Literature, the tables have been laid out in a horseshoe shape, all facing into the middle of the classroom. The backs of the chairs are almost against the wall, with just enough room to squeeze round and find a seat. This is new. It's bad. Why have they done this? Why make it harder? I need to sit at one of the ends of the horseshoe so I can get out if needs be. But the end over by the window already has a few people sat there, and I can't sit at this end by the door – which would've been perfect – because then no one else can get in. Why is barely anyone here yet? If I was a little later, maybe this is the seat I'd get, because the horseshoe would already be filled. Oh, shit. I should go back outside and wait in the corridor. But the handful of people already here, and the dumpy tutor, are looking at me. I'll seem weird. The tutor will make a comment.

Fuck's sake, I need to move: standing here like I've forgotten where I am is as weird as walking out. I sidestep between the wall and chairs, round the horseshoe, to a seat. As the classroom fills, I mentally rehearse how an escape would play out, and how much attention it would cause. The narrow gap between the back of everyone's chair and the wall is closing as the seats are pulled out from the tables to sit down on. The students rest their bags behind them, against the wall. I'd have to step between the bags, careful not to trip or crush something, and ask the kids now tipping their chairs back and leaning against the wall to move.

More and more come in. I'm being buried.

I draw down the margins of my notebook whilst our teacher sits an old stereo on his desk and hits play on a reading of *The Ancient Mariner*. Less than three hours until I'm home.

On the bus I listen to the rare second disc of Radiohead's *In Rainbows* that someone James knows put on a memory stick for us over Christmas. I now love disc one, so this has a lot to live up to. It's messier, louder, but I like it.

My stomach burns again, so I twist the Polo tube wrapper up and put it in my bag, hoping the nausea they keep away won't start up.

We leave Winteringham as '4 Minute Warning' closes.

I scroll through my iPod for what to play next. Click on Nine Inch Nails, but hesitate. Scroll up to LCD Soundsystem and try *Sound of Silver* again.

At home, the first thing I do is wash my hands. College and the bus are filthy. Getting sick would topple me from this highwire of good attendance. I reach for the hand towel, but stop when I think of my family drying their hands on it after taking shits, touching things in public, the garden. They wash their hands and effectively wipe all that crap onto this towel. I flick the water from my hands, go through to the kitchen, dry them on the tea towel. Surely that's cleaner, if it's used to touch cutlery and stuff. Plus I see Mum change them all the time.

9

A week passes, and another. I only miss one day, and despair when I do. I meet teachers to discuss the huge catch-up needed to meet the entry requirements for Huddersfield or Nottingham Trent University. Their references come through. I email each one a thank you. Those who taught me this year say I'm welcome; those from last year say "ok".

In the mornings I see the sun above the metal roof of the Maggy May, and plot where it will arc through the sky, how high it will reach this time of year, how soon it will set over the sports halls and the building where I go to counselling. Every day it must inch higher, and I must savour every day because tomorrow will be longer.

Sunday evenings develop a routine: run a hot bath, drink cold water, get to bed just after nine with a hot water bottle under the sheets, read a page of *Lord of the Rings* as my eyelids get heavy. It helps me feel prepared for the towering Monday morning.

I reach one hour fifty minutes at Emma's. We're at the dinner table again. My eyes return to the tub of melted butter, which slides off knives as it's transferred onto slices of white bread hung over the edges of the family's plates. Mashed potato slowly melds into gravy. They have bread and butter pudding for dessert, which I've never heard of. 'None for me just now, thanks,' I say, feeling my forehead tingle, starting to sweat. 'I'm okay for now, thanks,' I say again when Emma's mum offers me a cup of tea. We watch a traffic cop show in the living room and then I announce, 'My dad's probably outside.' Emma wraps both arms round me and squeezes. 'No he's not!'

The relief, when I see the car waiting for me.

Me and Emma cling to each other in the cold; the bus is late every night. When it arrives I catch myself feeling fond of its dusty warmth. In the long stretches between stops – where the doors open and nearly all the heat is lost – the throng of passengers and the brick-in-a-washing-machine engine get it pretty cosy.

Emma puts her little feet up against the back of the seat in front.

'How the hell do you do that?' I try to jam mine up there but don't fit. My knees are in my eyes and the effort makes the girl in front of us turn round. 'Sorry,' I say and settle for resting my knees against it. I mock smashing my foot against her seat again and Emma pinches me. Why does she do that? A flurry of gentle pinches and nudges. It always makes me laugh.

'Naughty,' she says.

'Nooty,' I repeat in her London accent.

We're on the top deck one night and the bus pulls over in Ferriby. I look down to the path and see a girl run straight over it, into the long grass between a crumbling brick wall and a fence, almost out of sight. Just visible enough to see her undo her trousers, jumping on the spot. She begins to squat down. I look away, and hope everyone else up here does the same. A minute later she gets back on and we set off again.

I get prescribed oxytetracycline – an antibiotic, for my acne – on a Friday. On the Sunday, Mum's lounged on my bedroom floor, turning the drugs' Bible-paper literature over in her hands whilst I play *Shivering Isles*.

'Well have you *had* diarrhoea?' Mum says, tipping her head towards me.

'No. But it's in the top five side effects.'

'You got these on Friday, and it's two doses a day. That's six doses by tonight. I think you'd have known about it by now.'

I slide off my chair and slump on the carpet. I haven't seen Emma all weekend in case that particular side effect suddenly kicks in. But what if the only reason it hasn't happened yet is because it takes a few days, and it'll all hit me tomorrow, on the bus or in college?

'Are you worried about the fifty *other* side effects?' Mum continues. I like it when she mocks my worry. It makes me know it can't be serious.

'Not as much.'

But I have read through them all.

Hang on: aren't most sickness bugs cured by antibiotics? Is oxytetracycline one of the drugs they use? In which case, taking these tablets every day is a kind of shield. An antibiotic shield. It will stop a bug taking hold before it makes me throw up or suchlike. This could be brilliant. I almost fact-check it on the internet, but perhaps it's best not to risk finding out that a thought so soothing is wrong.

I must at least be half-right.

A virus, though. Nothing can stop that. But keeping clean, avoiding sick people and being careful where I breathe is a start.

On a bus ride home, all the seats are taken but the side-facing bench near the front, where a guy's sat with a saggy old dog resting beside him on the seat. I dither about, thinking there's got to be *somewhere* else, and I can't stand all the way home when there's a seat right there: people will think I'm weird. The bus watches.

Emma sits on the bench and pets the dog, saying hi to the man. But she's on the *far* side of the bench, leaving a small gap between her and the dog for me to sit. For fuck's sake. I can't tell Emma to move up. I'm the man: I'm meant to sit between her and strangers. I sit down and look at the dog's flappy jowls spreading over the seat, just millimetres from the side of my leg. My leg muscles are tensed, just enough to notice, because if they relax, that tiny gap will be lost. Then later in the journey the dog re-shuffles itself, sits up and looks up at its owner, who gives it a little rub, his fingers slipping under those cheeks, into the raw skin and saliva. It lies back down, touching me this time.

Emma leans over and gives it another ruffle. She misses Perdita still.

She puts her hand on my knee, then finds my hand and takes it in hers. After touching that minging dog. I almost see the contamination spots on my jeans and hands. I want to rip my hand out of hers and say 'What the fuck are you doing?' but instead just stroke over the top of her soft knuckles with my free fingers, feeling like *this is it*: I'm going to be ill.

But remember: **the oxytetracycline**. A few dog germs won't be enough to break through that. It'll be okay.

At home, I wash my hands at once. Dry them on the bathroom hand towel to scrape off the "big bits" – the main bulk of germs – then I wash them again until the water burns and dry them on a kitchen towel. I throw my jeans and top in the wash, get in the shower. I tilt my leg to the side and drip a blob of shower gel directly onto the section of skin the dog was leant against. Is shower gel enough to get rid of dog germs? I wonder, whilst rubbing it into a lather. After I've cleaned the rest of me, I still feel that thigh needs extra attention, so give it a second wash.[8]

The following morning, I'm surprised to find myself waiting at the stop outside my street, not ill, not skiving. The bus crawls up the hill in the dark and I get on, into the warmth. We pass by the fence I used to hop, and Top Field beyond. I am that grid of yellow-lit windows in the dark that I used to turn round and watch go by.

At weekends I make music, knitting together samples into long ambient washes and dance beats. I upload a couple of tracks onto Myspace and Ben comments beneath, *No way did you make this. If you did – fuck!!* I keep looking back at the comment, wishing his approval didn't make me so damn happy.

Dad watches an F1 race in his chair. I'm on the sofa with my laptop. I lean into the microphone below the screen and in my thickest Yorkshire accent say, 'Jacket tatey,' and manipulate the recording, looping it over and over. Shifting the pitch up like a mouse squeak, down like an ogre, stretching it and compressing it, making it echo endlessly or reverberate, as though it's being said in the centre of a grand cathedral.

It's not until I hear a wheezing sound that I turn and see Dad wiping his eyes; his chest shakes with laughter under the cushion he always lays over himself.

'What the hell are you on?' he says.

---

[8] In a reality TV show where contestants trained like the SAS, there was a part where a drill sergeant stands bollock-naked in a tiny paddling pool and has the budding soldiers form a circle around him. He shows them how to wash when out in the wild. He uses his fingernails to scrape dirt from his legs. I wonder whether I should try this now, but then imagine how the germs from that dog would get rammed under my fingernails, where they might remain and multiply despite me trying to wash under there. Sometimes, does washing only move the germs? Does the water just dilute the filth, spreading it over your body, gathering it between your toes in the base of the shower, rather than completely wash it away? Does washing muck from your body only work it into your hands?

10

Nanna walks in whilst I'm at the kitchen table, arranging photos of fog and snippets of writing into my Art portfolio.

'It's working, that stuff. Whatever you're taking.' She nods.

I touch my chin. 'Really? The doctor said it'd be six weeks before I saw anything.'

'No, I can see it. You're clearer. Less red.' She hovers her hands before her own face, as though pretending to put cream on. Nanna always shimmies her hands about when talking.

That it is clearing my mild acne is almost beside the point. Oxytetracycline protects me from illness. I think about it when I eat a mint at college without washing my hands[9], when I unavoidably touch a door handle that thousands have touched only today[10], pick up a coin I dropped on the floor, flick through a second-hand book in class, hold the yellow bars on the bus if I've got to stand in the aisle.

At night I thank God I'm able to come to college now. When things get really hard in the day, I might pray to make it through to the evening, and apologise for asking, since my desperate prayer was sent back in Florida. "Nothing can stop me now" and "We're going in straight and true!" repeat in my mind as I traipse down to the bus stop, across the courtyards to my classes. I think of the Eminem track 'White America', where he aggressively shouts "I'm *lovin'* it". The sickness gurgles under me and I get through the day in spite of it, saying, *Bring it on, I'm* lovin' *it* in my head.

I think about Devon and Surrey: how to break it to Mum and Dad that there's no way I can go.

'Isn't he looking better? His face,' Nanna says when Mum comes in, too.

---

[9] After deciding that washing my hands in college's bathrooms will probably contract more germs than not bothering at all.

[10] Who have each touched a thousand things that a thousand people have touched, that have been touched by a thousand people, who have each touched a thousand things, and so on.

Mum trots to the side and re-flattens the clingfilm on a couple of the bowls of food she's got laid out. She takes a large black tray from the cupboard and arranges the bowls inside it, ready to take down to Grandma's. She nods to Nanna with a polite "Certainly!" smile, and glances at me.

'Are we actually moving to Grandma's?' I ask.

She shrugs. 'It's a balancing act, Christopher. Grandma and Granddad can't do some things now. They're getting on. But it's a case of needing to be ready for us suddenly having to be there. Granddad's not steady on his feet. I can't suggest helping with certain bits because they won't have it. You wouldn't like someone coming round and telling you how to decorate your house, or suggesting that doing this or that is too much for you.'

'Is that a "no"?'

Those ancient objects everywhere, radiating a… sickness. A curse, almost. Invisible but present.

Decades-old dust. On my fingertips, in the fabric of my clothes, floating in the air.

Out of date food in the cupboards.

'I don't know,' she answers. 'Bring this tray, will you? It's a job getting it in the car.'

'I'll make myself a cup of tea,' Nanna says.

11

It must be weeks since I listened to Nine Inch Nails or watched porn. At night during a prayer, I ask, 'Is this right? I'm trying to be a better person. Not what I was last year.'

I've been able to go to college, and I couldn't before. This might be what the problem was: I was blasphemous. Asking for God's help, whilst being a shit person the rest of the time. Look at last autumn: it started feeling wrong to play Nine Inch Nails or watch porn, but I ignored it. And it got me more and more sick.

In fact, that's stupid. Certain music and videos making someone housebound?

But can I risk it? He might take it all away from me. Leave me where I was before Christmas.

There can't be any exceptions.

Sorry, my mind wandered, I say to God, and continue my prayer. I thank him for looking over me whilst I go to college, for giving me the strength to see Emma more.

12

Emma goes home early and I spend the afternoon looking forward to listening to my iPod on the journey into safety. But Sebastian finds me waiting on Glover Road, and I know this solitude is now replaced with an hour's murmured monologue about music, Stanley Kubrick, politics and extended *Family Guy* quotes. And above the bus's engine and everyone else's chatter, I barely hear a word he says. I have to fill the gaps in between what's understandable, laugh when his voice suggests a joke, lean away from his halitosis.

We leave Winteringham on the thin tractor's road. A girl comes past me, says something to the driver, and our bus pulls over. The doors *pisssh* open and she dashes out. Is that the same person as last time, going for a piss again? Or something worse? A minute or two later she gets back on, smiles and raises her eyebrows at her mates at the back as she passes Sebastian and me. I hold my breath until she's well behind us, until the bus is moving again and hopefully some air has circulated in here.

Only a few hours until it's time to take some oxytetracycline.

I get off at my stop and breathe the freezing air, relish the darkness. Walk up to my house, wash my hands and dry them on the back of my trousers, where my calves are. It should be clean material there: it's a part of the trousers that don't really touch anything.

At night I sign off MSN but keep chatting to Emma via texts. She's asking whether we'll live together some day.

When I go to bed, my phone does a little buzz every few minutes, reminding me of a text I haven't opened yet. It's comforting, as though Emma's with me without having to be here making me nervous. I drop to sleep.

13

It's February. A no-man's land between the long nights of winter and the full foliage of summer. The sun's out of sight when I get home at night, but the sky is coloured, the streetlights still asleep. It's light in the morning, and as we curve down the hill into Ferriby, or trundle between the long hedgerows, I try to spot opening buds on the knots of grey twigs.

The panic keeps down, like, I don't know, something buoyant chained to an anchor. It would rush up to the surface of the water and spring out. But the chain's holding.

I pray not to be how I was. I try to be good.

The hot flushes, the squeezing stomach, they don't come as often, and when they do I close my eyes and ask God to help me – on the seat of the bus, in Emma's bedroom.

And when I feel sick, I ask, *Why did that happen?* What have I done wrong in the last few days that I haven't begged forgiveness for? There must be something. The scene in *I am Legend* I watched where Will Smith snarls, "There is no God. *There is no God,*" perhaps. Listening to the Radiohead line, "God loves his children." The track 'Lake Somerset' by Deerhunter, where the bass line's all menacing (which might be antichrist) and the lyrics are obscured under noise and distortion; they might be saying something blasphemous that I can't hear. I should Google the lyrics. Something's slipped through the net. Ben, in his garage loft bedroom, ranting to us all about the self-contradicting stupidity of Christianity, and I nodded. Not because I agreed, but to acknowledge I was listening!

I decide it's best to only play *Bioshock*, with all its themes on religion, when there's nothing to do the following day. In case, as with food poisoning, the punishment for playing it comes the following morning. On a Friday night, I'll think I'm free to play it; on a Saturday night, I'll feel a little less free; on a Sunday night, it's an absolute no.

One morning, I step on the bus and say hi to the driver I had a go at to impress George when college first started. He doesn't seem to remember me. Does he get so much shit from his passengers that my little attempt didn't stick? Will I be punished? It was a year and a half ago. But I feel the offence I caused stuck to me like muck, and want to introduce myself and apologise.

'You alright?' Emma says.

'Yeah.' I sit down. 'We've got the Goblin driving again.'

We're surrounded by people play-fighting back here. One of the boys jumps across the back row's laps. They try to pull his jeans down and roll him off; he flicks his shoes from his feet, onto the couple sat in front, who jump up with the shoes in-hand and wipe the soles on his pale t-shirt. A girl I went out with in primary school who apparently got bummed in Year Eight does a throaty shout and squeezes a jet of Powerade at someone. The lad falls into the footwells and pulls a guy down with him. He curls up as he gets slapped with the shoes he flicked off.

Emma nudges me out of a daydream.

'Kiss?'

14

I wash my hands when I come home, I wash them if I touch garbage, the rabbit hutch or Bentley himself, any object in the garage, the garage door[11], my Xbox controller, particularly if a friend

---

[11] Due to my family being in and out the garage for tools when gardening, touching the handle with a muddy, composty hand. And when I clean Bentley's hutch, I go through to fetch straw and sawdust, touching the handle with hands that may have been touched by rabbit waste, despite my best efforts. These days, I try to open the door with my elbow, like a surgeon, but the handle's so heavy that I bruise my arm and often drop whatever I'm holding.

has used it[12], the TV remotes[13], the carpet, living room furniture, my shoes, my belt[14], my nostrils, old objects, objects relating to my grandparents. When I'm out and about and wash my hands in a friend's sink or at college if it's desperate, they don't feel clean, and I make sure to wash *that* wash from my hands at home.

And often, even at home, one wash doesn't do enough.

Dirt can take two or more washes to completely get off the skin, so why shouldn't germs? Stood by the toilet sink, as I turn off the hot tap and flick the water from my hands, I still feel dirty, feel the need to wash a second time, so I pump another puddle of soap into my palm.

Hand towels still don't feel right. If I use a towel that I realise is a little damp, or isn't clean, and has effectively re-dirtied my hands by using it to dry them, I will re-wash. The backs of my jeans below the knees become permanently damp when I'm at home, sometimes wet-through. But if I remember my shoe brushed the back of my leg earlier today, or the back of my leg was against the chair I was sat on, or if a stranger's satchel may have touched the back of my leg but I can't be too sure but can't risk it, I'll re-wash my hands and look for a better way to dry them. Usually I traipse through to the kitchen, my dripping hands hung limp in front of me, to dry them off with kitchen roll. Surely that's quite sterile. But even then, I turn round to go back in the toilet and repeat the process anyway.

I prefer washing my hands in the kitchen sink, away from toilet bacteria.[15] The Fairy Liquid feels strong and harmful to germs; I pour it neat onto my hand and scrub it into the creases of my skin.

Mum has a go at me for using up the kitchen roll, the scrunched soggy clumps of which often fill the bin.

---

[12] Thinking back to any recent illness they or their family have had.

[13] Which Dad touches whilst picking his nose.

[14] Belts, buttons and zippers are the first thing you touch after wiping your arse.

[15] But you must be careful not to let the soapy, infected water from your hands drop onto any dishes or cutlery in the sink.

'Why don't you use the towel in the toilet?' she says, stood by the hob dropping mint[16] into a pot of boiling potatoes.

I lean round her to pull the tea towel from the oven door handle.

'Don't want to.' I scrape the water from my hands in the patterned towel. Fold it and hang it back up. 'The towel in there's all dirty.'

'I changed all the towels this morning. How can it possibly be dirty?'

It doesn't matter.

'You're that bothered about hygiene, yet you'll wipe your dirty hands on the towels we use on dishes and knives and forks?' she says.

The more I think about things that are dirty, the more things I realise are dirty. It's like a world's opening up to me. And I **have** to keep clean; I **have** to keep going to college.

When I was eleven, we studied *Boy* by Roald Dahl. I remember the bit when a young lad, quoting his doctor father, argues with an adult that there's no point washing your hands: the world is so filthy that trying to be completely clean is a waste of time.

I remember things like this, which might inspire me to stop bothering to keep clean. But I also remember stories like Mark Evans, who "couldn't reach the toilet in time" when he had the shits, so his mum told James. I witnessed Fern Marylyn wet herself in primary school. Or more so I witnessed the laughing circle we formed around her, until she buried her face in our teacher's skirt, and through teeth that grimaced with dismay, narrated her own misery: 'Everyone's laughing at me.' The accidents children would have in primary (or even secondary) school would instantly define them. Add a barrel to their name. I felt sorry for Fern, but wondered how the teacher could stand there letting a piss-wet girl cling to her.

From being that age, I've been funny about the traces of other people's saliva and touch. Their... essence. If someone took a bite from my food, I couldn't eat it anymore. Mum would make

---

[16] That she snipped from the plant pot in the garden. Did she check for aphids? Was it from the edge of the plant pot, where Bentley sometimes stands up on his back legs to chew on them?

a child-appropriate curse and call me "Anti-Septic Anny", taking away my plate. James would say, 'Oh, sorry, have I *infected* it?' if he was the perpetrator, and I'd be furious.

But that would come and go. In secondary school, I'd drink from puddles, eat rose petals and raw crops, Ant's second-hand spoggy, spoggy levered from the pavement, paper, small amounts of gravel. Anything you dared me to do. I never washed school's invisible filth from my fingers before eating.

Today, to save my hands from direct contact with dirty things, I use my feet for tasks like shutting the toilet lid and pressing down the handle to flush it. If there's a pair of my socks or boxers on the floor, I anchor a big toe on it, stretch the other four toes forward like a pair of scissors opening, then pull them back across the floor, bunching the fabric up with them; my second toe presses against the nail of my big toe, the fabric trapped between them. Then I can move the item to the wash basket, hover my foot above it and spread my toes to release it.

There's a punnet of grapes in the kitchen on a Saturday morning, and I use my lips and teeth to pluck them from their stalks[17] because my hands don't feel right after cleaning out Bentley's hutch, even after three washes.[18]

'Well that's handy,' Mum says, appearing behind me.

I jump, embarrassed that I was caught acting this way.

'Jesus, you'd hit the roof if you caught one of us doing that.'

But it's working.

It only has to be until college is over. There's about four months left, then it won't be this way at all. When there's nothing to do the next day, my hands can be as dirty as you want. Like on the Friday night a couple weeks back: Emma was down south with her family or wherever so I didn't have to see her all weekend. Three whole nights until college the following Monday. I barely washed my hands at all.

Until Sunday.

---

[17] Not too many though. Never eat too much fruit.

[18] Two consecutively, then a dry, then a third wash and a dry.

I'm managing five days a week, now. And every lesson. Even the stupid General Studies AS Level that Umbridge/Thatcher insisted on me taking. A thousand of us sit in the main hall and different teachers struggle to get their clip-on microphone to cooperate as they slowly waltz across the stage. During a talk about science and society, a Chinese guy next to me stops his note-taking, leans over and whispers, 'Excuse me. What is "testicle"?'

'No idea,' I say.

If I miss one lesson, or a day, it gives the disease space to creep in and establish. That's why Monday mornings are so hard: I've had all weekend to think about Monday morning. And that's why it's all the harder to come back to college if I skip a day. Or to see Emma if I put it off for a while. It's the pattern I couldn't get out of before.

15

In Art, we study human form. A group of us sit around a big rectangular table. Portfolios overlapping each other's, sketching pencils of varying softness, pastels, watercolour tins and brushes getting passed between us. We shape miniature wooden manikins and sketch them. I'm the only boy on our table. And boys are what the girls talk about, before turning to me and saying, '*You're* a guy, is this what guys do?'

'I don't know what *all guys* do,' I answer. 'We don't have group meetings.'

They laugh.

A girl opposite me who sits straight and wears an army jacket, her long hair pouring down its front, takes the three sciences alongside Art, and says Art is the hardest. I must tell Ryan and Ben this later. She holds up a sketch she's made of me whilst I was busy talking.

'I missed him obviously, but it was more the stuff we did,' the group's ringleader continues. '*Every* Friday night, we'd do something. He'd come over and say, "Let's go ice skating," or, "Let's drive into Doncaster and see what's happening." And when we broke up

I was just sat at home doing fuck-all and bealing all night every weekend. My parents were like, "You've got to do *something*. Where are your friends?"'

When have I ever taken Emma somewhere? What do we do? I go over to hers, barely holding it together; we watch TV with her family or go up to her room and talk, cuddle, shag. Emma doesn't ask for more. And I can't give any more.

At the end of the lesson, our teacher hands out forms: sign up and pay a small fee for a nude model to come in.

Is this okay? Can I do this?

It's not porn, it's nudity. It's art. Education. I'd be sketching her and learning to draw humans better, not wanking under the table.

Either way, I would be stuck in here for – I check the letter – two hours! If I needed to leave, it's not like I could run out, open the classroom door, whilst someone's stood starkers in the middle.

Who would stop me?

The girls are making jokes about it all. I do a smile.

A sharp wind pushes against the doors out the block. Cold air rushes in and hits my face as I shoulder the door against it. There's a frost in the shade of the buildings; the pavement's dry where the sun touches. My personal tutor from first year crosses right by me, who I sent the *I don't want you to think I'm just skiving* email to last year when my attendance started going downhill, and who I managed to squeeze a prickly reference from in January. I say hi. He meets my eye but doesn't say a thing.

It's gone half eleven: I should be okay to eat something.

Rich first years congregate near the food bar of the Maggy May, kicking up a football, palming their hair into shape and straightening those bright tees they wear with the massive writing. To get food, everyone has to squeeze through them. Fit girls get eyed head to toe; ugly girls get murmurs and shouting laughs; delicate boys on their own get tripped on an extended foot. What a cliché. They barely lean a degree away when I say 'heads up' and sidestep through, buy some chips and find our table down by the glass front.

These are the first chips – the first warm food – I've dared to buy here since, when, autumn 2006? Surely chips can't harm me. They are mass-cooked, submerged in insanely hot oil; they are only potato.

I pull a chair over from an emptier table and join Ben and Ryan.

'Weey, Three Musketeers,' says Ben.

'Three Muskers,' says Ryan.

I blow on a chip and put it in my mouth, hopefully not letting on the massive leap this is for me, that this is the victorious result of an extensive internal debate, covering every scenario of illness and retreat. Now that I'm opening myself up to food poisoning and stomach upset, what sins have I committed that will knock down this weakening defence?[19]

My tongue instantly seems to melt to accommodate the tang of salt on the chip's skin.

I tell Ben and Ryan what the girl who does science said.

'*No* way,' Ben says. 'She can't take the sciences very seriously.'

'It's what she said. Art's the hardest.'

'How's it hard? "Draw a swan!"' Ryan puts on a flouncy voice. '"*Be* the swan."'

'There's a shit load of work you've got to keep on top of—'

It's no use: Ryan's Art teacher impression has them both laughing, nudging each other. Anger warms my skin.

After lunch I climb the stairs to the counselling room. Knock and greet Pru, inside. As always, when the door shuts behind me, a fear makes itself known. I'm very aware of where the door is, where the nearest bathroom is downstairs, and as the fear threatens to rise, I re-consider for the thousandth time today every other step between here and home, and every branching, branching, branching possibility of the journey. Would Pru understand if I left? Would I explain myself, or grab my bag and run? As I place my bag down, I make sure it's within reach. Look through the blinds: only four hours until nightfall.

---

[19] I shouldn't have lied to that Chinese guy...

We run through my progress. Pru suggests I have my next session in a few weeks' time.

'I'll email your deputy head and let her know how well you're doing,' she says.

Umbridge/Thatcher: I'd almost forgot this was all for her.

'What are you thinking about Devon?'

'Nothing's changed.'

'Do you think you could get a car by then?'

'No chance. I could never afford one, even if I passed my test by then, but that won't happen either. My Dad takes me out to practise, but I haven't had any lessons.' And I still don't know how I will manage those.

When I emerge at the bottom of the stairs, I see the room I met the nurse in, when the first mention of my problem set a lump in my throat. It seems like forever ago. These first weeks of term have stretched into a lifetime. I head the opposite way, down a few steps into the lobby, where the low sun makes the big glass entrance glow orange, and the floor blaze too bright to look at.

Our last lesson's Media Studies. Our tutor warns us that for the module we're doing on censorship, we're going to be watching some disturbing, racy and controversial films. I watch the conifers dissolve a little into twilight, but not dark. Today's Friday, which I'm still not used to. A Friday, and I'm here at college.

My family order a takeaway from The Surma, our local Indian. But I know I'm off to Emma's later, and Indians are renowned for giving people the shits. Even if I've never had that problem, tonight could be the night.

'I'll eat mine later,' I say when Dad arrives with the bag and Jordan is peering in, taking his box of curry out before Dad's even set it down.

Mum and Dad frown at me.

'Why?' Mum says.

'I'm just not hungry yet. I'll definitely have it later. Once I'm back from Emma's.'

'Suit yourself,' Dad says, throwing his keys onto the side and pulling his coat off. 'I see you've already sorted your own plate and knife and fork out, Jordan,' he calls after Jordan, who's already piled his dish up and gone through to the living room.

I play *Ratchet and Clank* upstairs until Dad's ready to take me to Emma's.

It's half seven, and as we leave Barton I enjoy the dark that reaches all the way to Hull, turning fields and the river into nothingness.

After prattling about a Media Studies essay I'm submitting, I mention meeting Pru today. It's disappointing that no one's asked me about it yet, but I've given up waiting.

'She said near the end that there's no point meeting up for a few weeks now, since I'm coming in so often.'

'Don't think I haven't noticed,' Dad says. '*Fight* it, Chris. This thing you've got.'

'And she's off to email the deputy head. The one from that meeting before Christmas.'

'Good, good. Keep fighting it, boy. Hey?'

He grabs my leg and rattles it to and fro.

'Yeah. I am. I always was. It's just different now.'

* * *

Dear God, thank you for helping me tonight. I was really worried. I know you're looking out for me when I don't feel good. Sorry if I forget it sometimes. I feel stronger knowing you're looking over me. Both tonight and every day. Thanks so much for helping me go to college again. Forgive me for anything I may have done to offend you. I don't mean it. Sorry, I don't want to make this all about myself. It's a selfish way to be. There are people so much worse I should be thinking about. Please look over my family. My parents who work so hard for all of us. Mum working until so late with horrible people and then taking care of us boys, too. Dad being at work by four or five and working so hard he falls asleep at home before he's had like a sip of tea. Keep James safe in Nottingham and Jordan safe at home. Amen. And all the people far worse off. I shouldn't have said "horrible people" who Mum works with; some of them are probably really nice. Sorry. Amen. And Emma – please look out for Emma. She's the nicest person I think I've ever met. She deserves to be happy. Even if it's not with me. But please give me the strength to make her as happy as I can. Amen.

16

Is this happening?

I prop myself up on an elbow and look about in the dark. My room, the world, is shaking. It carries on beyond all doubt: I'm awake and this is a little earthquake.

Minutes later Dad opens my door.

'Were you awake for that? That was an earthquake!' he confirms.

I settle back into my covers and think how nauseating that could have been. Like trying to sleep through that ferry trip across the channel when I was ten which made me vomit. Like trying to read whilst in a moving car.

Don't be stupid.

In the morning my stomach's empty as ever. But tucked away in that space – a little gas cloud, a heat shimmer – I detect a sickness. The earthquake, it might have rattled a motion sickness into me that's lasted through the night. It might have massaged a stomach bug into fruition.

I'm lying over the armchair by the window, my feet scrunched into the radiator. I take a sip of water without swallowing anything; it soaks into my lips. Its cool texture is slightly soothing, washing away the sickness. Jordan's coffee smells strong. Mum lies on the sofa under a brown throw; she often spends the night down here. Then I remember she's off work today, and it's like the day has a safety net being set up underneath it. She'll come get me if I'm ill, I hope. The TV shows images of the earthquake, the minor damage it did.

'Where's Skull Lady?' Emma asks as we sail by the bus stop she used to wait at.

'Don't know when I last saw her,' I say.

Emma looks at me with the corners of her mouth turned down.

17

College pauses for half term. The six or seven weeks since Christmas – they feel like I've tried on a different life to the one before, seeing if it fits. It's a time of awakening I already feel myself departing from. Spring's nearly here.

Half term was meant to be a cue to let myself unwind, let my guard down, at least until the last couple of days. But I don't stop washing my hands every time I go out the back door[20], touch my jeans below the knee[21], touch anything in my old room where we stored James's stuff[22], the piano[23], the sofa.[24] After a piss I close the toilet lid and push the chain handle down with my foot, wash my hands two or three times.

The skin on the back of my hands turns wrinkled and dry. The swirls of my knuckles are swollen. Red cuts appear in the little folds of skin, which open and sting when my fingers curl to make a fist or hold something. The delicate webs between each finger are pale,

---

[20] Which is touched after one of us takes the rubbish out and touches the wheelie-bin or green waste bin, after anyone comes home from work with the day's germs festering on their hands.

[21] In case my hand strayed into jean territory I use to dry my hands. Drying your hands *scrapes* the germs from them, so there must be germs lingering on the shin of my jeans.

[22] 'It just came over me out of nowhere!'

[23] Scum/granules between the keys. Oldness. Not to mention the piano stool.

[24] Dad's flicked bogies may well land on it. And the cushions he keeps on his lap whilst picking his nose or re-arranging his junk will be there. Grandma was sat on the left side of it last weekend. Nanna tends to sit on the right and talk about diarrhoea, or an old folks' home she visited to cheer up a few people before coming here and sitting there without changing her clothes.

collecting crumbs of dead skin and developing red cuts of their own.

I apply Fairy Liquid neat and scrub my hands together, lacing fingers between each other, rinsing under water so hot I yank my hands back and prepare for the momentary but agonising throb of a burn.

Emma comes over; she jumps onto my bed and tells me they might be getting a new dog. I tell her not to lie the wrong way round on my bed. 'I don't want your feet near my pillow.'

As half term goes by, I hope that having a week off isn't enough time for that *way I was* to settle back in, time for worry to rehearse its shows of terror that keep me from leaving the house. But on Sunday, I run a bath, read *Lord of the Rings*, fill a hot water bottle before bed. Say my prayers, in case any wrong-doing I've done today has slipped by un-apologised for. In the night my feet itch, and I dream we're going back to Florida.

By morning, I'm nervous but prepared. There's a glowing sky over New Holland when I look down the hill for the bus.

18

Mum loads up four dishes with a pork chop, runner beans and chips over by the stove. It's lunchtime on Saturday. Dad volunteers to bring them over to the table; I watch where his thumb hooks over the plate. Food in that vicinity can't be eaten. I turn the plate so the invisible thumbprint faces away, and part any remaining safe food away from it.

It could be worse. There are occasions when Dad's thumb touches an item of food, or dips a few millimetres into my gravy. A wobble of anger will go through me. That's it. Dinner's written off. 'Why aren't you eating?' I'm asked. But no one would understand the truth.

Usually I offer to take the plates across. My hands are clean. When I see Dad start picking up the plates, I'll reach between him and Mum to grab whichever portion looks like mine before he can touch it. And why does he carry drinks glasses by the rim, where my mouth is meant to touch? I twirl the glass, looking for his fingers and thumbprint; if I can see it, I keep it facing away, if not, I'll not drink at all. Asking for another glass raises questions I can't answer. And even my diversion answers get prickly remarks from my parents.

When we eat bolognese, chili con carne or jacket potatoes, we have a bowl of cheese in the middle of the table to sprinkle on our food. Dad's fingers make a fairground claw, descend into the cheese bowl and close around a handful of gratings. Mum and Jordan then take from the bowl and I shudder inside.

* * *

James's train arrives in the afternoon. Dad picks him up from the station and I'm here opening the front door when I see the wobbly image of The Hummer pull in to the drive.

'Letting the cold in…' Mum shouts from the living room.

'They're here,' I call back, and go out to the drive in my socks. 'Alright.'

'Now, then.' James grins, hoisting himself out of the car. As we go inside together, I catch the smell of liquor on his breath, or from inside his coat. He must be having so much fun.

I make a round of tea. Mum tries to extract everything about Nottingham from James whilst Dad cycles through our Freeview channels, his feet scrunching alternately on the tapestry footrest.

When we're alone, I ask James about the nights out again.

'Nothing's happened. Not really.' He frowns at the ceiling in thought. 'It's not like before, when we all had—' he leans behind him and closes the door, so Mum, who's now frying onions in the kitchen, can't hear, 'when we had student loans to keep us going. I'm *miles* into my overdraft. Like, at the limit. Apart from the one meal a day uni does, we've been living on tinned food. So it's usually just a flat party. Getting wrecked on the cheapest shit there is. A lot of us are actually knuckling down now, or just too broke to go out. But then a lot have carried on. The rich kids. You know. You can feel a kind of rift growing.'

'Is it loud when you're in your room, like, when you're actually trying to sleep?'

'There's a guy in our corridor with a massive speaker system, and my bed kind of jolts with every beat, even six doors down. It's fine with me, but his neighbour right next door – this real quiet, reclusive sort of person – got so mad, he drilled through the fucking wall. He had a drill! And the hole was right near where the guy's head would be if he was in bed.'

'Surely the hole doesn't help muffle the music.'

'No, and they can see into each other's rooms, now. It's awkward, really.' He munches down on his dunked biscuits, holding them vertically to his mouth. 'You not coming to Grandma's?'

Jordan comes home from rugby and everyone leaves for a while. I'm not sure why I didn't want to go to Grandma's. Maybe it's since we're off for a pub dinner tonight and I pictured their house's particles getting up my nose, into my mouth, resting on the wetness of my eyeballs before being blinked into my body.

I sit at my desk and scroll down a bunch of images to print off for my Art portfolio.

It would be so easy to visit a porn site whilst I'm alone in the house. Search through the bouncing, pushing, pulling, opening, penetrating flesh until I find something that makes me want to come. Click past a moment too graphic for me. Browse from video to video, succumb to each alluring thumbnail, skip through the video's timeline to find an act so astonishing my dick could blow up in my hand.

A little buzz, a need to stretch, a gentle tense, on the insides of my thighs.

A big sigh. I lean back from my work.

There can't really be any connection between watching porn and being sick, not being able to go anywhere.

Do you want to risk it? After how well you've been doing?

Oh, I don't know.

I re-organise my jeans over my boner, and wish it would go away. But it doesn't. Hot and pulsing, it needs attention. I can't work.

I find a video.

The camera looks down from the man's perspective. The woman sucks his cock, works it with her hand whilst kissing the side of it. She looks up to the camera. I skip forward. She's bent over. She's doing the work: pushing her arse back onto him, again and again. All viewed from his eyes. Her big, amazing arse fills the screen. The muffled sounds of a fake orgasm. Her back arches and bows, taking him in from different angles. Then the man suddenly thrusts, too. Taken by surprise, her hands grasp for the bedstead to stop from being pushed over. Ripples travel up her butt cheeks to her waist. Her arse claps against his hips.

I close the explorer window. Shut the laptop. Go through to the bathroom and come into tissue. And even as I'm coming, the excitement falls away, leaving the naked realisation of what I've just done:

Broken the contract. Betrayed the promise.

Sin. Blasphemy.

The weeks of blessing, courage, health: I've spat in God's face.

Time must rewind. I *must* take this sin back.

I'm stood[25] with my dick shrinking in my hand. I close the tissue and flush it away, clean myself up and go back into my room. Lean against the wall, then drop down into a crouch. Clutch the side of my head and close my eyes.

---

[25] I would once have sat on the toilet lid to wank, since I don't enjoy being stood up much, but surely germs from inside the toilet crawl round the edges of the lid. Who would want to sit there?

'Sorry.' A whispered shout, the sort you hear actors breathe through tears. 'Sorry.'

James and Jordan return from Grandma's and hang in my room whilst I'm on the Playstation. We chat away and laugh at shit I do on *Oblivion*.

Inside, I'm praying.

I'm so sorry. I was so weak. So weak. I knew I wasn't meant to, but I did it anyway. I don't deserve your forgiveness. If you could ever find it in your heart to forgive me. I've learned, for good. I was weak. But never again. I was stupid. After all you've done to help. Please forgive me.

Monday's coming. Punishment awaits me when I'm on the crowded bus, in the middle of a quiet classroom. My stomach and bowels gushing everything they've got. When will he choose to do it? Will I see it coming? Or is the punishment that I'm now too afraid to go to college, and all the ground I've gained since Christmas is lost? That Thatcher will see my attendance fall again and kick me out for good? That I'll fall down that slippery pit and be a useless doley all my life? It has to happen. I've broken the contract. I was given strength and protection for changing my old ways, and I've fucking *chosen* to go watch porn.

Sorry. Sorry. Sorry.

The apologies are long, grovelling, repeated every moment I remember what I've done.

In the evening, we're getting ready for the pub meal Dad has booked. I close my bedroom door behind me, give my arse, balls and armpits one more dry with the towel and hang it round my neck.[26] I carefully

---

[26] The towel mustn't touch the floor. All the germs accumulated from years of feet treading into the fabric, of the hoover's dusty head gliding over it, will latch onto my towel. And if I then re-use the towel, it'll spread onto my skin, which may later transfer to my mouth, if for example I wipe my mouth with the back of my arm, or sweat at the gym and the towel germs gather in the bead of sweat that travels from my forehead to my lips. Or the re-used towel could directly touch an orifice, which would welcome the germs directly into my body.

open one leg of my boxers[27] at a time and step into them[28], sit on my bed and pull socks over my wet feet.

A feeling of joy and hope switches on inside: a light bulb's gentle glow in a sprawling black landscape. It grows and grows. Am I forgiven? Were the hundreds of apologies heard?

'Yes,' the feeling seems to answer.

The glorious relief of a sentence being lifted.

Don't run away with it. It's progress, but not a guarantee.

Thank you, I pray silently. *If this is you forgiving me. I* think *it is. But I'm still so sorry. Thank you so much.*

I sit here for a minute, feeling that glow widen. Outside my bedroom door I hear drawers and cupboards open and close, James and Jordan walking about, Mum and Dad shouting up and down the stairs to each other. I prop the door open and finish getting dressed: jeans and a dark, fitted t-shirt.

'I love this top,' I say next to James, looking into the big landing mirror. I stretch my arms out. 'It makes me look so... buff.' It's

---

[27] I've got those fitted boxers, nowadays. A-Front shorts. It's comforting to know that, should the worst happen and I shit my pants, it wouldn't just fall down my legs like with regular, loose boxers. These are tight round the leg. Like a nappy. I could run out before the smell permeates whatever room I'm in, find a bathroom, clean myself up. Emma thinks I look hot in them. I get anxious when I see I'm running low on clean A-Fronts, and the regular boxers await me at the bottom of the drawer. I feel comfort when Mum drops a pile of freshly washed A-Fronts on top of the cabinet for me to put away. And comfort when putting them on, like now. If I'm at college and things get tough, I might remember I'm wearing A-Fronts and actually feel a little better, or remember I'm wearing boxers and feel worse.

[28] My feet, even freshly washed, mustn't touch the inside of my underwear. Germs from the bottom of my feet will transfer into the shorts and transfer onto me. And again, my movements throughout the day might inadvertently move these germs to my mouth. Or the germs might simply wander up my arse into my intestines. If a part of my foot touches the shorts, I retract the foot and have to consider whether to throw them into the wash basket and try again with another fresh pair. Every image of illness and where I'll be over the next week tumbling through my mind. Mum has started to notice fresh underwear in the wash basket.

terribly arrogant and I never talk about myself like that but I just feel so good. God is forgiving me!

Crispy batter caves in under my knife. The fat chip on the end of my fork scoops up a thick dollop of mushy peas. James tells the table about an archeology dig he will be doing for a few weeks over summer. Mum asks whether living in a tent will make his perpetually stiff neck worse. Dad sips a bitter, sucks his top lip and bottom lip in turns, looking into the pint, then hands it to James. 'What do you reckon to that? Hoppy,' he says. Me and Jordan have a mouthful too.

'Very hoppy. Full of hop. Of *too much* hop,' I say, and Dad smacks me round the head.

Every few minutes, or is it seconds, there's the *knock, knock, knock* that I've committed a terrible sin today. Like happiness is underwater, and I keep surfacing for air and momentarily see the truth: I watched porn. Did it really happen? Her arse filled the screen, pushed back on his wet cock. I sought the ideal video out, clicked through link after link; I could've stopped any time. But I couldn't stop. That build-up to coming: you don't just get halfway and think, *okay, that'll do*. But I *should* have. I'm supposed to be better than that. I send God more sorrys. Because that good feeling may never have been forgiveness after all.

19

Like standing outside with my palms turned up, checking for rain, I spend the week wondering when the killer blow will happen, what narrow space I'll be in when I'm sick so hard my body whips about like that alley scene in *Team America*. But it doesn't come. Class to class, journey to journey, I wait for it, until I see the cement works' red lights on the Friday night journey home, Emma stroking my hand, and it seems like God really chose to be forgiving.

'Am I seeing you tonight?' she asks. 'I'm off away next weekend, remember. Unless you wanted to come.'

'Don't know,' I say.

Haven't I done enough?

The fear of retribution trickles through to the following week. But there's another suspicion then.

In the last year of school, I set my MSN title as '700', then every day when I'd sign on, I would decrease it by one: '699', '698'. I didn't know what I was counting down to; it was meant to be mysterious. Friends asked about it online, in the school yard. Sweet attention from girls I had a crush on. Classmates I barely knew would open conversations with me and ask about it, and the ice was broken.

MSN is less populated nowadays, and I don't go on it much. But today, the countdown finally hits zero. I text Emma the news before college. Then I rub styling gum into my hands and ruffle it into my hair.

My Motorola buzzes against my leg.

Ooh. What happens now?!!!xxxxxx Emma asks.

A thought occurs to me as I get on the bus: did I never know, halfway through Year Eleven, that I had begun a countdown to my ultimate disaster?

Boris bounces next to me on our walk down from Glover Road to the Maggy May, demanding I reveal the countdown's fruit. It's brought up at our table. Cartwright and Bethany drum their hands on the surface and interrogate me whilst the others smile and wait for my answer.

Ben sits down with a stack of toast and a bottle of full-fat milk.

'Oh God, the countdown.' He puts on the voice of an adoring fan: '"What does it *mean*, Chris?". "Now, now, ladies. One at a time",' he answers, as me.

'Shut up.'

The smell of buttered toast is amazing.

'Does it mean anything at all?'

In Literature, I wait for the feeling of illness that never arrives, whilst we listen to another reading of *The Rime of the Ancient Mariner* on CD that sends ripples of laughter through the group.

In Art, a girl has a drawing pin stuck in her sole. She takes the shoe off and picks at it, but can't get her fingernails under the pin's mushroom head. Touching the sole of a shoe! Our gossamer teacher, who I sometimes picture as only a head and hands holding up her flowing black dress, holds the shoe and turns it round in her hands. Then I'm astounded when the only other boy but me in our group, a big rugby prop with a little mop of blonde hair, takes the shoe and bites away at the sole.

'Ooh, don't do that,' our teacher breathes, her fingers to her lips, laughing.

He gets the pin between his teeth and pulls it out, the shoe jerking away from his mouth as it comes free. 'Tadaa!' he says through his teeth, then spits the pin onto the table and gives the shoe back.

How can he do that? He lives in Doncaster!

By the time the day's up it starts to seem like the countdown meant nothing after all, and that's a relief. The closest it comes to disaster is our bus taking another detour to the depot because someone throws up upstairs again. But I think about my oxytetracycline and send a prayer. Mum and Dad have the news on after tea; I go in to check if the countdown led to an event bigger than me: opinions about Prince Harry being taken out of Afghanistan; something about American politics.

20

Emma and her family go down south, and I spend Saturday excited to go to Ben's with the boys and have some beer. Without Emma, it doesn't matter how nauseous even a couple of tins make me feel later on. It's seven when I leave home and cross the roundabout, past the big hairdresser's house with the tall hedge. My fingers reach out to snap a leaf off, break it down the stem, throw the two halves away, as I have for years every time I pass, but my hand hesitates. *It's a small vandalism, and a disrespect of life.* The words are spoken to me from elsewhere, floating up from the murk of a shaken magic eight ball. My hand nestles back in my pocket.

A bunch of us cram into Ben's attic bedroom and drink. Toggs, a fat chav in the periphery of our friendship group who we haven't seen since school, flicks through Ben's yearbook, and like a stand-up comedian says something mean about every loser in our year. He makes a joke about Emma's "frog eyes", unknowing that I'm now with her. By the time I've formed a retort, the conversation's moved on and I don't know how to resurrect the subject. For the next hour I want to butt in or leave.

'Then look at *you.*' Morgan points to the Year Seven and Eleven photos of me. 'Who would've thought you'd turn into this intelligent, buff guy?'

I wake up from the angry daydreams and throw Morgan a flirty wink, whilst secretly touched that he noticed my distance and wanted to cheer me up.

We start making prank calls. I don't know how we got here, but Ethan's got his phone calling a random number, Ben's there with his laptop open, on full volume, his finger poised to hit play on a porn video. As soon as the voice of a poor old lady picks up the line, Ethan says in a formal, agitated tone, 'Hello, this is porn,' before the video blasts orgasm noises into the mouthpiece. And everyone blows up with laughter. We don't hear at which point the old lady hangs up.

Did I suggest part of this? It was a blur of escalating laughs. It may have been me. Even without knowing. Oh shit. I'm laughing but inside my goodness rots away. I'm sat in such a way that I can't see the computer screen, so I'm technically not breaking any rules, but this is **not good.** I'm disrespecting other people. I'm hearing porn. But the image of me turning serious and saying, 'We shouldn't do these boyish pranks that might upset other people, and you shouldn't watch porn,' is enough to make me cringe.

Sorry, I say internally. *Sorry I'm doing this. Should I leave?*

And I wonder whether everyone else here will be punished. In fact, how many people in the world watch porn?[29] How many people make prank calls? Are they punished? I'm thinking they aren't. They certainly don't go around throwing up and shitting themselves. The world would know; it would be a fact. Mothers would point and say to their son, 'Look at that man in front of us with the soiled jeans. That's what happens if you make a prank call.' Unless these sinners are punished in a different way, and don't know that the bad times they go through are because they watched porn or upset an old lady.[30] Or punished in ways *they* are afraid of: they lose money, prized possessions fall to bits, they get injured, for example. Surely we would all see the connection. And that's like me saying bad things happen to bad people. Which can't be true. When I think of people suffering cancer, and all the loved ones affected by it, are they all being punished? What have they done to deserve it? If I investigated and interviewed them all in their tortured state, would it turn up sinful reasons for the cancer?[31] If my family dies in a car crash tomorrow, should I assume they've all done one of the things I know I shouldn't? Or, shit, should I assume it's me who's being punished? Why do bad people get away scot-free? There are footballers and film stars who are wankers and live the highest life. Businessmen who have crushed partners, ignored their family and exploited the poor on their climb to the top, who live to a happy old age with a wife a third of their age. Why wasn't Hitler struck with illness up there in front of the saluting millions? Why are the band members of Nine Inch Nails, the creators of this music I can't listen to, out there touring, bathing in the crowd's adoration? Is their punishment lying in wait for

---

[29] As Dr. Cox said in *Scrubs*: "I'm fairly sure, if they took porn off the internet, there'd be only one website left and it would be called *Bring Back The Porn*."

[30] Making the punishment useless, surely.

[31] Would I even see the red flags, or are there sins I don't yet know are punishable? The family might seem innocent, the cancer a terrible misfortune, but the clue was staring right there at me. What don't I know is punishable? How will I find out? Will it be too late?

another time? Can I just not see that they are suffering? Will every member of the tens of thousands at *every* gig, on *every* tour around the world, be sick for enjoying that anti-religion music? I don't understand. It's like Karma. Karma that only applies to me. But that's not Christian. Perhaps this world is merely a staging area – God's elaborate dream, constructed solely for me. No one else is in this system of punishment because they don't exist. It's a test to see if I'm worthy of Heaven in the end. Everyone who meets in Heaven has been through their own dream-test. And it's only since Christmas that I've woken up to how it works. What should I think? I don't understand.

Sorry.

Toggs is telling one of his monologues.

'Nowt's worse, man. Standing at the bus stop before college and you got a shit brewing. And it's like, ah fuck. I gotta hold that shit in all day. Like ten hours. You know what I mean?'

He's told us one about holding shits in before, years ago. When we were thirteen. The story involved being on the other side of the Humber Bridge and suddenly needing to go. Telling his mates to go on without him and biking home like the clappers. It's echoed around me ever since. And even as he's telling this one, I know I won't forget it. I couldn't tell anyone a story like that.

I know what Toggs means. I've held in shits all day at college this term, until the urge to go fades completely. In the evenings I try to go to the toilet, then say to myself, *that's it for twenty-four hours, now*. It's distressing when I can't squeeze one out and I know it's a whole day until I can try again.

21

My portfolio's in my pigeonhole in the Art room, and I need it to finish my write-up about negative space. In a free period I go to retrieve it.

Weird. Why's the classroom door closed?

I open it.

Why're the lights off?

Oh.

Round the middle partition I see the naked woman in the middle of the circle of tables, a dim spotlight above her, and just within the rosy periphery of its light, the faces of the surrounding students, looking up and down from model to paper, as though making notes on a lesson her body is giving.

For the next day I wonder whether punishment will come for this intrusion, this invasion.

22

We watch the first film of our censorship module: *Death Mills*, a long-banned-to-the-public documentary about the Nazi Holocaust.

An orchestra chugs dramatic music. The narrator's voice hacksaws through the poor recording technology of the time. In a posh American accent he lists off the many ways in which millions of prisoners were killed. Slow starvation, poison gas, bullets and bayonets, suffocation in train carriages, strapped to operating tables and mutilated in waking experiments, crammed into furnaces, thrown amongst the dead and allowed to fade. We watch the faces of those the Allies found alive in dungeons, as they were gently led or stretchered into the light with faces marked with astonishment.

The Allies tread through dark warehouses of the dead with clipboards in their hands and pipes in their mouths. The immeasurable tangle of rotting humans form dunes and troughs, a landscape reaching beyond the camera's gaze.

In the daylight the dead are piled against buildings and walkways like snowdrifts. Skeletons with skin. They litter the ground, everywhere. One or two still move an arm or lift their heads – oversized now, compared to their withered bodies.

The Allies dig up the mass graves, autopsy the bodies. We see close-ups of gawping dead faces. Children and newborns shrivelled up like dead spiders on the soil. Adults carried around in the naked, starved state they were left in, hung like white rubber over the soldiers' arms, and I'm scared I'll see one fall to pieces.

With a forensic eye they study another warehouse which was filled with prisoners and set alight. A close-up of a man's head, shoulder and arm squeezed under its wall: he'd almost dug under it and out of the blaze. We see the camp survivors stood before a table of doctors, a stethoscope held to their back, their bodies agonisingly thin. Why must they be naked still, now they are free? A woman undergoes treatment, her hip bone exposed through a gaping wound. Survivors shuffle around in a daze, naked and skeletal. Image after image of wasted life. The music blares; the narrator's vowels are piercing.

The film ends and the tutor turns the lights on. It's the last lesson of the day. We talk and make notes, then I go down the stairs and into the windy evening. I sit on one of the courtyard benches, waiting for Emma. And I risk saying to God, *Why did you allow this?*

The question hangs in emptiness until I say sorry.

* * *

We study three controversial films from 1971, and the one we watch in full is *Straw Dogs* for its double rape scene, the first of which many argue the victim appears to enjoy. Attending the lesson might count as me wanting to watch sex – in a terrible form, no less – on a screen; but not attending the lesson might make me slip back into never attending.

It's for education's sake. Surely it's allowed.

I don't know.

In the opening half hour of the film, I try to look at the blank page of my notepad, though it's hard to stop my eyes glancing at the screen.

This is ridiculous: it's just a film. Just watch it.

So the rape scene approaches, the climax of a predatory tension between the female protagonist and a bunch of sweaty village workers. She finds one in her living room whilst the husband's away: an ex-lover. Her rejections aren't enough to stop his advances. He slaps her. He raises his hand, ready to hit again if she doesn't submit to him there on the sofa, so she does.

It turns into a surreal love-making scene. She moans in pleasure, reaches her face up to kiss him. This isn't right.

It's sexy.

No. Oh no. I can't be turned on by this. This is despicable. It's criminal.

'Sorry,' he says into her chest when it's all over. Sorry like I was after watching porn. Full of self-loathing, maybe.

Then the part we were warned about. A second man comes in, pointing a long hunting gun at the sweating pair on the sofa. Without words he gestures the first man to climb off. A little flick, flick, with the gun. The first man shakes his head, but moves aside and holds the woman face-down; the second man undoes his trousers.

Her "*no*" as it becomes clear what's about to happen crackles the speaker. Unlike the first rape, this is edited like a machine gun – a chopped-up mash of the man's thrusts, the woman's face scrunched in agony, covered in a sweaty tangle of hair. I flinch, look at the red walls beside the screen. The film's infecting me. I send thoughts of regret up to God, for lacking self-control, allowing my eyes to view the scene and not just stare at my notebook like I was meant to. But far, far worse, for momentarily seeing something erotic in that first scene. God, what am I? A rapist in the making. A rapist. Just kill me now. I'll accept whatever punishment you give to me, I say. I deserve it. I deserve it.

'Okay. There we have it,' our tutor says, hitting stop on the projector and walking past the screen towards the light switch. I sit forward in my chair, put an elbow on my table and my forehead in my hand. What's happened? What happens now?

23

Parents' evening is another spike on the calendar, sort of visible over there in the ever-shrinking distance, that I wish wouldn't get closer. At least this year I've told Mum and Dad it exists. Our first appointment is after six. This means going home only to immediately hop in the car and come back to college. So instead, I do what once would've been the unthinkable: stay at college longer than a full day.

Emma kisses me in the Maggy May and goes off to Glover Road. There's no denying it anymore: it's broad daylight at four, now. I watch students crisscrossing over the courtyard, meeting up or heading home alone. The herd thins. Here inside, there's suddenly only a dozen people. Then only me and a couple others, all throwing distance apart in this massive hall. I rest an ankle over a knee and sit back, open up some work, run a highlighter pen along a few lines of poetry, but I can't concentrate.

The bus will be gone. I've sailed off the edge of the map.

No one would know what this means to me: conquering college so well that I'll voluntarily stay for longer than I need to.

Fear rises and falls. Thoughts of being ill in this new situation surface and sink, like a volume knob's being tweaked up and down, demanding I watch the images with full attention when it's loud. But I'm happy. I notice the sunlight begin to saturate and watch the sky, the buildings, the people walking by, until it's a little fuzzy outside, until it's lighter in here than out there, until I can see the hall's double-vision reflection in the glass. The girl near the vending machines gets up, shoulders her bag and heads through the far doors. My phone rings: Mum and Dad are here.

My Art teacher calls me "the comeback kid". My Literature teacher says I've done a great job this term "in spite of everything". We chat to my personal tutor Neil about how things have changed since before Christmas. 'I'm dead happy for you,' he says, with a big toothy smile, crow's feet pinching his eyes.

We sail down the M180 in The Hummer. Me and my parents talk about the teachers' comments, about results and going to uni this autumn. I move to the middle seat at the back and put the belt round me.

'Have you heard back from the unis yet? With these "conditional offers"?' Dad asks.

'No. It's still early to be hearing back.'

'I think you're going to absolutely *love* it. God, I wish I'd gone.' I see his eyes in the mirror; they glance at me.

Through the windscreen, the cat's eyes – red, green and white – make a kind of runway home in the black. There is the motorway, and there is nothing.

When I go to bed, my feet itch and I keep them outside the sheets until I fall asleep.

24

'Come here, let me see,' Mum says.

I lay my hand flat on the kitchen table, beside my notebook. It's a Saturday morning.

She comes over and peers down to study it.

'Christopher,' she says, touching one of my knuckles with a couple of cool fingertips.[32] 'You need to stop washing. At least put some Nivea on.'

'Nivea only makes my hands all greasy and horrible.'

'Your skin's a barrier against germs, too, you know. If you keep making them drier and drier, you're destroying that barrier.'

---

[32] Should I wash my hands? Mum's always clean, I'm sure. But she's cooking dinner. She may have handled raw chicken. And even if she's washed her hands, a little bit might remain there. Like the symbolic germs and virus cells you see in disinfectant adverts that look like giant oscillating ice cream sprinkles. One wash doesn't get rid of them all. They linger on every surface. How many surfaces and door handles has Mum touched since she last washed her hands?

I've got no reply. I make a gentle fist and watch the little red cracks open.

Chicken's sizzling in the frying pan. Mum returns to chopping onions.

'You should wash your hands after the loo and before you eat. Not every five minutes. Are you even going to eat any time soon?'

'You never know. Or I might forget to wash before I eat.'

'I doubt that.'

'And there *are* other times when you should wash your hands.'

'Yes, alright. But you know what I mean. You're doing it too much.'

'Are you using the same knife for them onions that you did for the chicken?' I ask.

'Don't start on food safety with me,' Mum says. 'I've cooked your dinners since you were born. Have you ever gotten food poisoning? No. And it's not the same knife. I cut the chicken with these scissors, look.'

I go wash my hands.

25

The days get lighter; I cling to night time as it's pulled up away from me. I watch the buds of trees as we pass them and silently beg them to open. Then they do. Bit by bit, the naked bushes and trees' fingers start to fill. Not quite enough to hide inside yet. I think about last year's summer – the heat, feeling sick like Harpo, the ringing in my ears, squatting in that den under the bushes in the pouring rain, taking an energy drink to the gym that Dean mistakes for beer, meeting Bitty's dad down the farmer's track – and feel like it will repeat, like it's connected. The year cycles through seasons, therefore so must I. We're heading to summer, therefore my attendance *will* get worse, like last year.

You've done great through winter, though, I tell myself. You've broken the cycle.

It doesn't stop the feeling of a loop.

It's the same with music. I can't listen to *In Rainbows* without feeling its connection to the past. Like it's a tether between the **me of now** and the **me of last autumn**, and it's enough to pull me back there. I'll hit play on the bus, but it bombards me with images of trooping around Barton in the cold, watching the bus leave in the dark without me, wanking at home or playing *Halo 3*, frost on the ground, pushing pale, wet, naked twigs out my way as I walk a squelchy path through the woods, feeling afraid. And if I keep listening, the present will melt away, and I'll realise I'm still in autumn, still sick, forever avoiding everything.

A film might play on TV that I can't watch. Jordan puts on *Hot Fuzz* one morning, which I love and quote all the time with Jordan and Ben, but I leave the room. It's too connected to last summer – sweating, nauseous, pulling leaves off bushes, listening to *With Teeth* and *The Fragile* by Nine Inch Nails, not knowing the stains I was making in my soul. Five minutes into watching *300* I turn it off, because I feel the dark, central-heated nights of last autumn, the Sunday afternoon lethargy, the inevitable failure to escape Barton's fearful gravity, surrounding me, ready to be my reality again.

James comes home for the weekend and we talk about Radiohead whilst he scrolls through my iTunes library. When I mention how *In Rainbows* reminds me of when I couldn't go to college, he puts a fist to his chest and says, 'Did it help get you through some tough times?'

'No, I mean it reminds me of it too much. I struggle to listen to it.'

'Oh,' he says.

But "reminds me" isn't the word. Perhaps "takes me there", "threatens to turn me into the person I was at the time of first listening to it", "contains, and threatens to bring forward, the bad parts of me I carried at the time of first listening to it", is more accurate. Even though I talk to James about being nervous to go some places, I'm not sure he'd understand this. I couldn't explain how certain music, films, games, our piano, objects, even places, **carry bad things**: skins I could slip back into. I can't go back to Top

Field or Death Hill in case I breathe in the haze of **past** hanging over them and it re-infects me.

James clicks on Nine Inch Nails[33] and says, 'I've been listening to these, lately. I've got *With Teeth*.'

'How did you come across Nine Inch Nails?'

'You,' he says, with an "of course" tone.

It's my fault. I made him listen to 'Please' on full whack when he passed his test and we were cruising around town in Mum's Fiesta last year. I banged-on about how good *Year Zero* was and made him listen to those kind of electronic solos of 'Vessel' and 'Great Destroyer' in my room; he even bought me the CD for Christmas, which I haven't taken out the seal. He never seemed fussed about them. I didn't think any of my attempts to get him into them, before I knew the truth, worked.

Should I warn him what'll happen if he listens to them?

'How long've you been listening to them?' I ask.

'A while, now.'

A while? What's that? Since last autumn. I wrack my brains: has James mentioned being sick since he started listening to them? Has anything else in his life fallen to bits? It's too weird a question to ask directly. Our conversation carries on, seemingly normal I hope, whilst I'm wondering: does the misery just need time to take effect? Will it not be long now before James starts being unable to leave his apartment in Nottingham?

I introduced him, *persuaded* him, into this. What punishment will I get for coaxing my own brother into anti-God music?

It was before I knew, I say to God now. *I didn't know, these last few months, that he'd actually started listening to them. Please forgive me. I wouldn't have played him the music and talked about it if I'd known back then. I'm so sorry.*

Part of me thinks, no, don't forget it's only me who will be punished for listening to Nine Inch Nails. James, and everyone else, is alright.

---

[33] And for a moment I'm terrified he'll click play on one of the songs.

26

As I come into the bathroom for a shower, a stray corner of the fresh bath towel I'm carrying touches the carpet near the toilet. Or did it? Fuck's sake.

I lock the door behind me and turn the shower on. Fold the towel onto the wash basket. Tuck my thumbs under the elastic of my boxers to pull them down, but I don't. I deliberate whether I can do this: use a towel that's just brushed over a spot of carpet where specks of piss have rained down since we moved in six years ago. Six years of not hitting the bowl quite right with a stream of piss. I'm guilty of it. My brothers and Dad must be. What about friends who have come over and used the toilet? Sometimes, when I was younger especially, that first half-second jet of piss would miss the toilet entirely before correcting itself, and I'd tread a wad of tissue into the wet mark on the carpet. I can't be the only one who's done that.

Six years of build-up. I can't rub that on myself. Even if only an inch of the towel brushed the floor, it must be enough for something to transfer. I grab the towel and bunch it up, flash it under the shower to make it seem used, stuff it in the wash basket and get another, carrying this one more carefully. After I shower, I'm careful how I dry myself, that the towel doesn't touch the floor, sink, wall, door, shower curtain. The act of vigorous drying makes the towel flick out. I slow it down, make sure I'm in control. Then I throw it in the wash anyway.

I clean my hands. The last thing I wash is my arse; I don't want any residual germs from that on my fingers.

Mum soon notices the towels piling up in the wash and homes in on me.

'Are you just using a towel once, then throwing it in the wash?' she says one night.

I hit pause on *MotorStorm* but don't turn from the screen. 'Sometimes.'

'Christopher.' She lets her hands drop to her sides. 'I can't keep up with this much washing. I'm trying to put two loads on every night after tea. And sixty percent of it is yours. There's more wash-ing from you in a day than Dad in a week. It costs money. It's hardly fair. Is it?'

I don't answer. I can't re-wear gym gear. I can't re-wear clothes that touch a seat I don't like the look of at college, or get a few of Bentley's hairs on.[34]

'I mean, why is there a set of your bedding in the basket now?'

'It was dirty,' I say. James had propped the pillow up and lain on my bed to play PS3.

'It was fresh on on Saturday. Do you know how long it takes to dry bedding in this weather? Do you just throw anything into the wash and think, *Mum'll sort that. She's got nothing better to do?*'

There's a pause between each question that I've got no answer to fill. She goes away.

Later on I go downstairs for a drink. I open the dishwasher. Warm steam plumes out and wets my face. I take a glass and study it in the light. Run the cold tap and fill it up[35], pour it out, fill it up, pour it out.[36] Again and again, until I'm satisfied any dishwasher salt has gone and that the water is pure.

---

[34] I can't re-wear clothes that touch the sink as I sidestep into the downstairs bathroom; clothes I wear to Emma's; clothes that a stranger brushes against in the streets; clothes a fleck of dishwater hits if I'm filling the kettle and the cold water stream makes a splash in the bowl; clothes I wear to my grandparents'; clothes a tiniest dot of food touches, because food goes bad, and I can't carry bad food around on me, in case its germs seep into my skin or I touch them and then my mouth or food I'm going to eat; clothes that grass cuttings touch when Mum asks me to mow the lawn; clothes that touch either of the bins as I squeeze down the alley behind the house; boxers that touch my feet as I step into them; clothes I wear if I sit on the carpet here or in a friend's room; clothes I wear. Clothes that have touched clothes that have touched any of these things. Like, if I'm folding fresh clothes, whilst wearing clothes I know I'm going to throw in the wash tonight, and the new clothes brush against these old clothes, I'll scrunch that fresh t-shirt up and throw it back in the wash.

[35] Damn. Should have waited longer for it to run cold. This could still be a bit of the residual hot water going into my glass, or water left standing in the pipes.

[36] Even though I've rinsed it half a dozen times now, I still wonder if some of that first premature fill is left, even at an atomic level.

27

Emma wordlessly strokes my hand on a ride home I was so nervous for, I almost hid in college to avoid it. When we're nearly home, I take her hand in both of mine and kiss it. She turns from the window and smiles as though happy to see I've finally woken up.

28

My stomach feels uncomfortable. I think back to the last few days, the last few weeks – what I might have done wrong. If there's a punishment due. There must be something: I'm getting ill.

At least it's happening at home, not at college. God can't be that mad with me.

But it's a Wednesday evening: tomorrow I've got to face being there again, and I'm scared.

I daydream of urgently needing to shit on the long, slow, crowded journey in.[37] Situation after situation, pulled through my head like knotted rope.

Worst-case scenario, I'll take some of the tablets in my bag. But that would be admitting I have diarrhoea. Admitting that I'm desperate. Which makes it worse.

---

[37] The painful stop/start crawl of our bus, the volume of chatter, the watching eyes and word-spreading mouths. Emma beside me. The squeezing need inside my abdomen for a bathroom, for an obscuring bush or wall, a place to subtly call one of my parents to come find me and bring spare clothes. But how would that play out? I picture Mum or Dad's reaction when they pull up in the middle of nowhere and I emerge from a hiding place, open the car door and they see their seventeen-year-old son has shit his pants. Driving us home, would they announce their disgust or roll down the windows and pretend nothing's wrong? Would they make me sit on a plastic bag?

I go downstairs, take a glass from the kitchen cupboard, run my finger under the cold tap at the sink until the water feels icy. Carefully fill and pour the glass again and again. Then I decide this glass isn't right, take a different one out the cupboard and start again. Throughout the evening I drink water, pints of it, hoping this process is flushing away whatever sickness threatens to take hold. Then I make a hot water bottle, get into bed, shiver for a while until the covers warm up, and pick up *Lord of the Rings*. The discomfort is still there, but it's subsided, and I've only been to the bathroom once. It'll be okay, I tell myself.

On the bus ride in, I feel like I'm floating. The sensible part of me kicks and screams, but it's not in control of the body anymore; the body just gets dressed and walks out the door onto the bus, thinking, *We're going in straight and true!* and *Nothing can stop me now*. I shouldn't think that second one, anymore. Sorry.

There's a dialogue in the story I wrote, where the protagonist asks his friend how he can always be so calm, despite the danger they are both in. His friend says the best way is to pretend you're on rails: you're trundling along no matter how terrible you feel. You keep moving, even if you don't want to. He's a character I wish I could be.

We watch a risqué black and white film in Media, about a woman rising through the ranks of a workplace by flirting and sleeping with people. Giving men The Eye before the scene cuts out and the camera pans up the building she works in as she fucks her way to the top. There were two endings filmed. In the one we see, the man she actually falls in love with dies. It's meant as a kind of punishment: women can't progress through life this way. You will suffer for it in the end.

Still, even with a film this tame, I'm frightened. There's a bit where she and her friend get to ride a train because she sleeps with the guard, guiding him into a carriage with straw in the corner. Her friend, seeing what's about to happen, turns away a little and sings, keeping look-out. The idea of her glancing over whilst the other two have sex stirs a little excitement in me. And if that's the case I'm essentially watching a form of porn.

I sit here apologising to God whilst the lesson carries on, even as I contribute to the class discussion.

The wrongdoing sticks like tar that I claw at to get off me, but it only smears, gathers under my nails. Remember *Straw Dogs*? What a sick person I am.

I know I deserve it, if you choose to punish me, I say. *I don't know what to do. Should I have skipped this lesson? Walked out when the suggested sex appeared onscreen? It's barely a PG!*

Sebastian catches me on Glover Road waiting for the bus. It's too sunny for mid-March.

'Hmm. I thought you might want to see this,' he monotones. From his rucksack he pulls out a handful of laminated photos and hands them over.

It's me. Taken from up high in the Photography block. I'm walking across the courtyard. Like photos of a wanted suspect.

'Ah right,' I say, already knowing how the others will laugh if they hear about this. 'Why?'

He shrugs and carefully slots the photos back into his bag. Says something I don't catch above the trombone exhausts of rich kids' hatchbacks that bomb up and down the road, darting between the idle buses.

'It looks like I was on my way to Art. There was that chubby naked woman in there again who everyone was sketching, but I didn't fancy it so I worked on the other side of that wall.'

'If you want to draw a fat woman, just ask Emma.' Sebastian stares at me like he does, to wait for my laugh.

'I'll tell her you said that.'

'Sorry.' He looks at the ground.

It's me who breaks the silence and changes the subject. Somehow I'm not sure being mad at Sebastian works like it would for most.

29

The clocks change.

Main course arrives. I slip my shoes off under the table to cool the itch. Look over my shoulder, past the small takeaway queue, to see how much light falls on the street.

Was it ever this light after seven? How much worse will it get?

Sebastian's birthday has fallen on a Sunday: I should be in the bath right now, preparing for tomorrow. Me and Emma received one of his customarily formal invites to join him at the Surma with his weird mates.

Finch wears a skintight Ramones t-shirt with holes burned into it; he looks like ten minutes outdoors on a cloudy day would give him sunburn. Squatted on his seat and scratching his arms, he brags about being "balls deep" in a girl earlier today when Sebastian was trying to ring him. He makes a couple of weed jokes to the waiter, then nips outside to buy some more from his dealer. We get it – you smoke weed.

We split the bill and leave for Sebastian's place. I have to walk slow with Emma, her legs taking two steps to every one of mine. Any quick escape is impossible unless I abandon her. Sebastian puts Nirvana[38] on quiet and they continue drinking. I join Finch at a high wooden table, rest on an elbow and watch him work.

'I can never do rollies,' I say.

'Practice, matey. As with anything. Have a go.'

'Na, I'm alright.' I enjoy smoking, but I'm afraid to touch Finch's stuff. There's something dirty about him. When he speaks in my direction, I subtly lean out the way, picturing his waft traveling over and getting sucked up into my lungs.

He puts a pinch of tobacco in an open Rizla and pulls it thinner until it's the length of the paper. Opens the little zip-lock bag of resin and pulls a corner off. Crumbles the brown granules amongst the tobacco. Tucks it all in with his long thumbnails, licks the sticky

---

[38] I was worried it'd be Nine Inch Nails. Sebastian was the one who introduced them to me.

bit and rolls it up. Twists the end and pops it between his lips. I can make out brown fingerprints on his joint.

All the while, he tells me weed can be grown straight out of compost bags: just cut hundreds of little holes in the plastic and push the seeds straight into the soil with a finger. He describes the ideal places to hide your crop and how to check the buds.

I remember when Finch got his finger trapped in a chewing gum dispenser at school and the fire brigade had to come.

'Didn't you get caught growing it once, near the end of school?'

'Never grown it myself,' he replies. He brushes the flecks of spilt tobacco off the edge of the table into his other palm and drops them back into his tin. 'That might've been Baker. He grew it in Bonby woods.'

'That's it,' I say, trying to dodge the direction of his breath.

'Yeah his weed had something really, like, grassy about it. Made Sherborne whiteout one time. I get mine from just round the corner from Surma, like you saw. He sells to cops and teachers. But it's not the same in my case. I kind of *have* to smoke mine because I've got Irritable Bowel Syndrome, and this helps.'

What the *fuck* is Irritable Bowel Syndrome?

I can only assume you shit a lot, given its name. Fuck's sake. He's been breathing on me all this time and passing himself on. I need to walk out, to breathe fresh air.

'It's proven to help. It's a muscle relaxant,' Finch finishes. 'And I can tell this isn't what you want to hear because you clearly can't stand to be near me.'

'No, not at all,' I say, shocked he picked up on it, and said it aloud, so politely. I notice how retracted my neck is, how far away from him I'm leaning. 'Carry on.'

'Nah that's it, really. Just…making an argument!' He holds up the joint. 'Now if you'll excuse me, gentlemen, I'm off for a smoke.'

God, I'm horrible. How many people have I shrivelled away from, who don't have the backbone to point out that they notice it? The scratters who sit beside me on the bus. Teachers who lean over my work, going over it with me, whilst I subtly cover my mouth and nose with a hand and pretend to assume a thinking posture.

30

Mums giving me a lift home, I feel really poorly. Sorry I wont be here xxxxxxxxxxxx

I read the text from Emma under my desk in Literature.

Poorly? What kind of poorly? Do I feel it too? I mentally pat myself down.

It's too close in here, the air and the sound. I can't reply, but spend the rest of the lesson feeling increasingly sick.

Awww that sucks. Whats up?xxxxxxx I type once lesson's over and I'm heading through the courtyard.

'Did Emma go home?' Boris asks in the Maggy May.

'Yeah. Didn't she feel well this morning, then?'

'Emma's always ill,' he declares. He said those exact words before me and Emma got together. I remember it making me worry that she was a sickly person who would pass things on to me.

But "Emma's always ill" doesn't narrow down what her current illness is. Would Boris be so calm if it was a sickness bug Emma had erupted with? No, he probably wouldn't be freaked out at all. He would've said something, though. It would've been the talk of the group.

Got a really bad headache.wish you were here to gently hold me xxxxxxxxxxxx

Thank God.

Headaches aren't tied to diarrhoea are they? They might be. But I'm pretty safe. If I get a headache, I'll just calmly march into town, get on a bus and go home. It's okay.

Sorry, I say to God. *I shouldn't thank you. Please watch over Emma and make sure she's okay. Amen.*

A couple of lads carry a water-filled condom the size of a small child from the bogs and gently lay it on a table near the entrance. Its blobby mass slowly stops wobbling until one of their group spanks it.

In Media we watch a clip from an old film where prisoners are force-fed shit.

Our teacher rolls up the blinds and the conifers out there sway in the bright sunshine. It's not so bad. I think about the ride home on my own.

When Media's over I close my notepad, still wondering what "This is", penned on the front cover, could've meant. Sometimes I see "This is" and in my head answer, *Yes, it is.*

I walk up to Glover Road and find a spot along the garden walls to sit against that doesn't have moss or fungus growing on the damp brick or concrete – wouldn't want that seeping through my jeans and boxers.

Sophia's alone, facing the road with her arms folded. She twists round and spots me, and I can see what she's thinking. She crosses the half-dozen steps between us, eyes scanning up from the ground to meet mine at the last moment, the way she would always approach.

'There's no need to look so terrified.' She smiles.

'I'm not terrified.'

'No, you're not. *Shit.* I can't believe we haven't spoke, all this time. How *are* you? How's Emma? Is she not here today?'

'She's fine. She just went home early, but yeah she's fine.'

'Because weren't you on a different bus before?'

I think how many times it's been Emma waiting here alone, or with Sebastian.

'I was just finding different ways back. You know.'

It's alien, to speak to her this way. And see her eyebrows move with exaggerated interest. Like colleagues. Everything we already know about each other is kept behind the gates. I want to talk forever, and at the same time don't want to talk to her at all; I want to stop the conversation and ask, 'Can't I talk to the real you?' But feeling like that's my business is what drove us apart in the first place.

Sophia had a theatrical silliness that could level me with laughter whilst amazing me how imaginative she was. And I could be stupid, as though with James and Jordan. We'd talk and talk and laugh; it was meaningful or ridiculous; it was always easy. And there's no going back to it. We're both making a display of maturity. I'm only grateful she hasn't witnessed how I've turned out through college.

'You guys seem really good together. Emma's like the happy pick-me-up to all your brooding,' Sophia says.

I pull a face. 'Well, thanks!'

And she laughs.

'She's certainly—' What's the word?[39] '—cheerful, which is refreshing. Have you got a special man in your life?'

'I'm seeing this policeman at the moment. He's thirty, which is a bit sad. But he's alright. I've been messing about too much and not knowing who the fuck I am and this is helping with that.'

'Sounds nice.'[40]

And on it goes. Excruciating, but I don't want it to end.

'I'd better leave you alone,' she says at last. 'I'm *going* to find you and pester you around college, though, so be ready for that.'

'I'll be ready.' I smile.

She goes and stands at the kerb again. A couple of her friends are there now. I dig my iPod out, take my earphones from their little case and hang them round my neck. I can't put them in until I've said hi to whatever driver we get. Ignorance must be one of the sins. Scrolling through my music, there's starting to be a few marked albums I can't listen to.[41]

---

[39] Be careful: a lie is certainly punishable. Don't choose a word that isn't true.

[40] What is it Liam Neeson says on the *Kingdom of Heaven* advert? "Speak the truth, always. Even if it leads to your death." And what is it Ned Flanders' kid says on that old *Simpsons* episode? "Lies make baby Jesus cry."

[41] The *Fight Club* soundtrack Sebastian gave me last year, because, one, it reminds me of last year; two, the film *Fight Club* makes numerous unholy claims; three, the track 'Medulla Oblongata' opens with a beat that sounds too similar to Nine Inch Nails' 'Me, I'm Not'. *At War with the Mystics* – I heard that before Florida and it makes me think of blinding light and a sedimentary nausea in my throat. And it was a wet morning in the first weeks of college, walking past the sandwich shop near Spar, that I heard *Through the Windowpane*, but that was kack anyway. Nothing by Muse, Pure Reason Revolution or Ray LaMontagne feels right anymore. I'd put *The Information* on, but it's got a track called 'Nausea'. I can't listen to *Bodysong* after being briefly hooked on 'Milky Drops from Heaven' last year on the many early journeys home, but the *There Will Be Blood* soundtrack is safe enough.

31

Emma's alone. Her family have gone down south but she's decided to stay up this weekend.

Its getting so windy. Am worried about the tree comin through the wall. Can u come stop over and keep me safe?xxxxxxxxx

A nervous feeling tightens my legs muscles. Do I feel sick? Is my stomach okay?

Dunno if Im sleepinxxxxxxx I reply.

Mum drives me there. I've been enjoying how windy it is all day. It's comforting. Now it's betraying me.

'I'll text or ring you then if I need picking up.'

'Yep.'

'So, assume I'm staying *unless* I text you. In fact,' I say, the momentary courage vanishing, 'can you come at eleven?'

'Right.'

My hair whips up when I step out the car.

The massive tree in the neighbouring field that arches over Emma's house is losing the still composure expected of something so thick. Its limbs lean back in the wind then throw themselves forward, bringing the whole tree with them, the branches bend, the twigs vibrate and lash about.

When I touch the gate, I make a note to wash my hands. I use as small a surface space of skin as possible to do the latch. The very tips of my fingers on only one hand.

Emma's wearing Ann Summers gear. I know it as soon as she opens the door in a dressing gown. She unties the rope and opens it for me to see. My heart flutters. We kiss here at the bottom of her stairs. My hands run over the red silk; her knees give and we laugh into each other's mouths. Emma hangs the gown over the banister and walks me through to the lounge.

Though my boner chafes against my jean buttons, I'm also weighing up whether this sex will mean I have to stay the night; I'm counting hours and minutes until eleven, comparing segments of time with other difficult things I've achieved; I'm hoping I don't become ill during the sex.

Later on, we cuddle on the sofa and laugh at some bonkers *Smurfs* dance track on TV.

'I'm making a brew,' Emma announces. 'Want one?'

'Go on then, please.'

'Fucking hell, really? Are you feeling alright?' She laughs.[42]

It's only Emma here. A cup of tea can't harm me. Think how many I have at home, and don't have a reaction.

But this house is dirtier. The fridge where the milk's kept is dirtier. The cups probably are.

What an appalling thing to think.

I watch the clock move through to half ten and text Mum for more time. She rings me.

'I can't come any later, Chris. I've got to be up first thing tomorrow. I was already asleep before you text me.'

'Okay.'

'Are you not staying there, then?'

I get up and go into the hall. 'I don't know. I don't think so.' Barely a mumble.

The big tree's twigs scrape on the wall.

You should be staying, something says.

Mum sighs. 'Right, I'll come at half eleven.'

That's hardly late, but I feel bad for dragging her out, and bad for not staying with Emma. Life would be easier for them both if I just stayed. James stays at Bella's for days; she stays in his flat for days. How does he do it? What happens when one of them needs the toilet? I don't even piss here at Emma's, no matter how much I need to.

'Thanks a lot,' I say. 'See you soon.'

Mum hangs up.

---

[42] A bad question to ask, because it reminds me that I haven't asked myself that question in at least thirty seconds.

'What's happening?' Emma asks when I emerge into the lounge again.

'Mum's getting me at half past.'

'Okay.' She smiles. The smile of someone hiding that she wishes I was staying. Or the smile of someone pretending to hide that she wishes I was staying.

She's quiet and shrunk. Emma might be playing a game to make me stay, or she might genuinely be worried to be alone. Either way, it's working. For the next hour I bounce between *the right thing to do* and the safety of being shot of this place.

As it gets to quarter past eleven, I go into the hall again and call Mum, but hang up before she can answer. Squeeze my eyes shut and tap the phone against my forehead. She'll be on the way – I'm committed. I'm letting Emma down, when she's frightened and alone.

My phone buzzes.

'What's wrong now?' Mum says on the line.

'Nothing – didn't mean to call you.'

'Right, well I'm setting off now.'

When I see the Fiesta's lights outside, I say bye to Emma, who asks if I will text her at least.

'Of course,' I say. 'Fuck's sake.'

'What?'

'Nothing. It's just me.'

I kiss her and step outside.

Wind rushes over the black field. The metal fence wobbles, the clumps of grass on the green blow flat. Twigs and leaves scratch along the pavement. I shouldn't be leaving.

'What is it?' Mum says when I open the car door but don't get in.

I watch the tree waving back and forth towards the terraces. I duck down and say, 'I might stay,' into the car.

Mum turns away, hands still on the wheel.

'Sorry. Emma's just on her own, and not really comfortable – with, like, the tree…'

'Are you staying or coming?'

Watch the tree again. Look at Emma's front door, where the security light's still on. She must be back in the living room, writing a text about wishing I'd stayed. But the morning is a long, long way away. And the more angry I make Mum, the less chance I have of someone coming to rescue me in the early hours.

'I should stay.'

'Right.' Mum's staring out the windscreen. She turns to face me. 'Well close the door then.'

'I'll text you in the morning.'

'Mm hm.'

She turns the car round and off it goes.

Is it too late to stop her?

A single streetlight looks down on this little car park; the green and the row of houses hide behind the dark. The sound of Mum's car fades to nothing. I picture where she'll be by now: taking the right onto the main stretch out of Barrow, towards the sixty road, probably picking up speed sooner than she should. How would she react if her phone buzzed now? No, I'm stranded.

Emma's blurry image comes down the hall. She opens the door. Glances over my left shoulder with an inquisitive frown. Ready to look relieved, if the absence of a car means what she hopes it means.

'I'll stay.'

As the time creeps past midnight, past one o'clock, my Lilo drifts too far out to sea; I can barely see the shore. I wonder whether I can feel a shit brewing.

We go to bed. I open the window even though it's cold out; Emma shuts the bedroom door even though we're alone.

She puts on a silk nighty and jumps under the duvet that's piled up with clothes. I lie next to her and hold her body in my arms. Like any other time we cuddle.

Let yourself go to sleep for once, I tell myself. No need to stay awake and tell Emma it's time for me to leave.

I feel that distant stirring in my belly. Do I need the toilet? Can I wait until morning? I'm frightened that if I go to sleep, I'll shit the bed. I need a piss, too. No, I can't go to sleep. I'll lie here and keep guard. That's what she asked for, after all.

Emma keeps shifting. She's awake, too. A little shuffle, and another. Whenever she does, her arse, through that silk, rubs over my cock. She moves it up and down against me, so slowly it could well be in her sleep. Her cold thighs and cheeks drive me crazy, knowing how warm she is inside. My dick's hard even though my mind's far from in the mood.

She gives up and falls still. I've no idea if she's asleep. I just track the slow progression of the shit inside me, inching toward the gates.

You're fine, just go to sleep.

I can't. I can't let my guard down.

It's only Emma here. She's kind. She'd keep a secret. What is there to be worried about?

I watch the teal digital clock on Emma's stereo. Speak prayers in my head. Wait to see any light come in through the curtains, constantly wondering how much I need the toilet, if at all.

Emma lies perfectly still. I'm convinced she's still awake, until she farts twice, rubs her cheek on the pillow and brings her knees up a little higher.

My six-thirty phone alarm goes off, and though it's the Easter holidays now, I get up, put clothes on, send a text to Mum.

I've made it through the night, fighting to keep awake, listening to Emma breathe and watching each minute on the stereo clock, but this must count as our first time sleeping together.

Be there at 8 en route to work x Mum replies.

Jesus, another hour and a half? I don't think I can wait much longer.

Emma gets up, too. Sleepy and confused. 'But we could lie in.'

'I'd rather be up is all. You can sleep. I don't mind.'

'No, it's okay,' she says.

I make us a cup of tea and we sit in the lounge not saying a word. BBC Breakfast plays on TV, and I watch the minutes change on the clock at the bottom corner of the screen.

Half an hour before Mum comes, I give up waiting, go to the upstairs toilet and take a shit. It's a green colour. I'm as quick as humanly possible, so Emma hopefully thinks I only went for a piss.

32

It's the heat. Obviously it's the heat. As soon as my feet are outside the covers, they stop their wretched, prickling itch. It's these Sunday night baths I can barely lower myself into, the hot water bottles.

But I've heard that last year, James had a scabies mite on his feet. It kept him up night after night, tormenting with a terrible itch until he figured out what it was. And then his girlfriend Bella fucking told everyone.

'What did James take when he had that scabies thing?' I ask Mum one morning.

'Some lotion,' she says, in between the kitchen and garage. 'Why?'

'I just worry I've got it.' It's taken a while to gather the courage for this conversation, so I'm not holding back now.

She frowns. 'Why would you?'

'How would I know why?'

'It's just so rare, Christopher. The chances of even James getting it were small. I doubt you'd get it, too.'

'But my feet itch every night, so much. Couldn't they live in the carpet and then I tread on them? Since I'm in his old room.'

'I really don't know. I doubt it.'

'Was there any left over? Any of the lotion?'

'Probably.' She roots in the back cupboard in the utility. 'Yeah, there's still some here.'

When no one's home I take it upstairs and read the label.[43] It says you should even rub it into your groin. I can't shower for twenty-four hours after using it. Right.

I get seeing Emma out the way that night, before lathering my feet in the lotion. My toes lace into each other to work it in; I keep them off the floor until it's dried. Then I rub the lotion into my

---

[43] Even if touching the bottle means any mites left on it may scuttle over onto my hands.

hands, burning all the little cuts on my knuckles and the webs of skin between my fingers. White and creamy, it smells like polish. It says to reapply each time you wash your hands. There wouldn't be enough even in a full bottle for that.

33

A new Leggott Porn circulates. Not quite porn like the last, consensually filmed one. This time, a guy walking through the car park across the road notices a Vauxhall Astra rock on its suspension. He starts filming on his phone, walks up to the car and there they are: a guy and girl going at it in the reclined driver's seat. They don't notice their spectator, who after five or ten precious seconds knocks on the window and shouts 'Weey!' or 'Busted!' and they scramble into defensive action, shielding their faces and crotches, trying to pull their clothes on.

At least this is how I've gathered the film goes.

I could never watch it. Cartwright asks if I've seen it yet, getting his phone out, but I say 'Yeah' and laugh like I'm remembering it. In Media before our teacher comes in, two people are leant over a phone with it playing on loud. The phone's lying right there on the table; I can see the colours glowing out the screen. I study the red wall, the steel window frames. I draw a kite in my notebook.

There's a three-hour lull before the bus home, since I no longer leave early even on days I actually have a free afternoon – I can't give the illness an inch.

The shadow of a window transom creeps over the circular table in the Maggy May, where I'm drawing highlighter lines through photocopied handouts. I place a hand on the surface and keep it still for half an hour whilst I continue taking notes with the other, occasionally checking on the shadow as it advances in a line diagonal to my hand, beginning with my forefinger's nail, eventually covering my little finger, all my knuckles. The sun's still moving, even when the days are long.

Emma and Boris come in from Biology. Boris is even more hyper than usual, which is funny until he suddenly grabs my yellow high-lighter and stuffs it in his mouth.

'Give it back, you minger,' I shout-laugh, whilst furious inside. Like an excited dog, my protests only make him happier.

When he puts it back on the table, I already know I'll never use the highlighter again.[44] But it's in a pack of four. I can't put it back in the pack, because his saliva will transfer onto my other pens.[45] But I can't *not* put it in the pack, because Boris or Emma will ask why I've left my highlighter pen here on the table. They wouldn't understand the reason. What can I do?

'It's ten to,' says Emma, getting up.

I wince inside.

Just think of the oxytetracycline that awaits me tonight.

Resolving to note every part of myself I touch between now and when I wash my hands at home in an hour's time[46], I put the highlighter in its packet. I'll simply have to buy a new set. I use the fingers that didn't touch the highlighter to carefully put my work back into my bag. As we walk out, I know Emma will take my hand; I move to the other side of her so she gets the clean hand.

---

[44] The pen has landed overlapping a sheet of notes about the nationwide Festival of Light. I can't touch that again. At least, I must remember the top inch of the page that the pen has come into contact with and never touch it. Nor the top inch of the other sheets of paper that this sheet will have to come into contact with inside my bag. Second-hand transfers. I must sear the pen's position in my mind. I *mustn't* forget and touch that part of the paper.

[45] And onto my hands when I next use the pens, and into my mouth if I eat without sufficiently washing my hands. Boris is never poorly, but mouth bacteria is mouth bacteria. And who's to say he won't be ill tomorrow? And this saliva harbours the dormant virus/infection?

[46] Including every piece of clothing I touch, which will be thrown in the wash.

34

Pru doesn't turn the heating on. She in fact mentions how mild it is today. We're going in straight and true.

'Everything's fine, still. I'm still unsure why.'

It's because God looks over me. Because I've changed my ways.

'Excellent. You've been to, what, most of your lessons now?'

'No, all of them. Since we last spoke, I haven't missed one. It's extremely hard. You know. And sometimes it's even harder than that. But if I miss one, I feel like I'll fall backwards. It's like...' I splay my fingers and squeeze the air, '...like it's a muscle. The more I fight against this nervousness, the stronger I get. And if I *don't* do the things that make me nervous, the muscle might get weaker, less used to fighting, and the things that make me nervous will seem all the harder next time. Does that make sense?'

'It does. You treat keeping on top of this anxiety like a form of physical fitness. The more you fight it, the better you are at fighting it. But you've got to keep "fit" by fighting it all the time. It's a nice way to put it.'

'Exactly.'

'Now, last time we spoke, you were still concerned about a couple of things. Your exams, and your family holiday.' She taps her biro on her fingerprints as she counts the short list. 'Both of which aren't all that far away, now.'

I fill my cheeks and blow. 'I don't know. What to do about. Don't know.'

'Pretty daunting then, still?'

'Yeah.'

'College was daunting though, five or six months ago, wasn't it?'

'It still is.'

'Yep,' she nods. 'But you manage. You seem to manage more every day. Is it so far flung to imagine you'll keep managing more, over the next month or two?'

'I guess,' I strain, not convinced.

'You've got your repertoire of the last few months to call upon. Think of the hard times, and how you overcame them.'

I've prayed, and tried not to do anything wrong. And overcame things by *just doing them*. That's my repertoire.

'About the exams, though,' Pru says. 'Students have been known to take exams at home, when they are unable to attend the hall or room or wherever the exam is. I believe you have to be watched by an invigilator, who'd come to your house. People with varying disabilities go down this route, but I think you would qualify. If you think this would be good for you, then you should get applying soon.'

She'd think I was so sad if she knew how much I just lit up inside, hearing this.

'Maybe. I'll see what they say in student support, shall I?'

'I can write you a reference. So, in truth, I think we've been through all we need to go through. I'll write to your deputy head again and let her know about your progress. You've done a remarkable job. And I think you'll continue to. Remember, should you have a relapse, a relapse is all it is. It doesn't mean you're going backwards, and it's all part of the journey to being better.'

'Yes,' I say, a little worried that we're coming to the end of these sessions.

'And don't stop bearing it in mind, like you have been doing. Perhaps this nervousness you feel is just part of life. You feel nervous coming to college, well *I* feel nervous getting on a plane and being launched up into the sky. When I was young, I would be absolutely petrified of flying. My fear luckily ran its course, and then it faded entirely away. For decades. But then my husband and I were on a holiday in New Zealand. We were about to come home. And our little plane, for some stupid reason, just halted in the middle of this scorching runway and the pilot said we'd be there for twenty minutes or so. And just like that, I remembered *I'm terrified of planes*. And I absolutely panicked. I wanted to jump up and escape the plane.'

'Sounds horrible.'

'My point is, I wasn't ready. I'd let myself forget how bad things can get. Fears don't tend to *go*, you just get them under control. If

I'd given a bit more thought during those occasional flights I went on in those years without panic, maybe that panic in New Zealand wouldn't have happened.'

35

I throw the pegged-out washing over the top of the line so it's out my way[47], pick up the bird table[48] and put it to the side of the garden, move the barbeque.[49] I mow the lawns, and it makes me sweat.

'Look, Mum.'

Mum's shearing round the edges of the grass.

I show her the inside of the grass bag, where there's barely two handfuls of clippings. 'What was the point?'

'It still neatens it up.'

Bentley runs round and round the old football, pushes it along the edge of the grass, then climbs onto it and humps away until it drops down into the mud. He stays still for a moment, wondering what's just happened to his lover, before hopping down to sit beside it.

---

[47] I should have washed my hands before touching the washing. Especially this bath towel. If I end up being the one using it, and all our bath towels look the same so I'm as likely as anyone else, I'll be rubbing the muck that's on my hand right now – that's transferred onto this towel – onto my body.

[48] Carefully holding it by the post, but the table itself touches my forearm. The bird table! Where those filthy birds eat and shit. Where their scratchy little feet that have been who-knows-where skitter about. Shit, shit, shit. I must remember to scrub this bit of arm. No, get a shower. No, scrub the arm, then get a shower.

[49] No doubt even the handle still has some remnant of last summer's barbeques. Meat juices, left to age. Remnants of **last summer** rubbing onto me. There have been frosts since then. Surely that's killed the germs. Killed the germs? Would you eat a pork chop that had been left outside for nine months just because it froze over once or twice at some point?

I open the recycling bin and tip the grass bag into it. The way the air swirls inside the bin when a new load is tipped in makes the tiniest sediments of grass plume out the top. I step back and bash the bag against the edge of the bin with one arm extended, but the little dots of grass land on me, and stick to the sweat on my skin. You may not see it, but it's all over me. In my hair, too, I bet. I blow through my mouth and spit on the floor, predictions of Monday accelerating. On the packed-mud ground, I spot the shrivelled up and darkened orange peel from when I sat on a bucket down here on that freezing morning, the winter before last.

I put the mower away and wash my hands three times until the water burns and the steam touches my face. Go upstairs and shower.

'My counsellor was saying you can have exams at home,' I say, sat by the kitchen table with a cup of tea and chocolate roll.

Mum snips the bottoms off flower stalks near the window. She lays them on paper towel. Rips the top off a sachet of plant food and squeezes the syrupy contents into a vase of water. The plant food swirls in the middle of the water and dissipates. Mum snaps round, with a downward-turned face. It means "you what?" for when one of us say something odd.

'People with disabilities, or the kind of thing I've got, can apply for it.'

'And how does that work?' She puts the flowers into the vase and starts positioning them individually.

'I think a guy comes and watches over you. You'll have to do the exam at the exact time everyone else does, still. So you can't cheat. He'll be like, "Start now," and off you – what?'

Mum's laughing.

'Christopher,' she says. 'Come on. You've done so well getting into college recently. Is an exam really so different? You're honestly saying it's better to organise some *Ocean's Eleven* bouncer to come stand above you, there at the kitchen table?'

I smile and try not to laugh. The whole thing sounds ridiculous but it's a way out. Come to think of it, having someone come here, with all their attention on me, might be just as hard. Would he stand at the door of the toilet if I needed to go in there, like Bella used to with James? Would he have to *come in with me* to check I don't text a friend or pull notes out my arse?

'It's your gig, at the end of the day, Chris. But I think you'll be fine without.' Mum rinses her hands, wriggles her fingers into the sink as though symbolising rain to a deaf guy, and wipes them on her gardening jeans.

It's been two weeks. Time for the second application of lotion.

Dad's traded in The Hummer for a BMW. Six years old but in beautiful nick, except for the crinkled driver's seat. In the evening, we speed out of Barton. He hurtles past slower cars that get in the way, turns to me and laughs, saying 'Jesus!'

He tells me again that he's proud of me for managing college, and how jealous he is that I'm going to uni.

'I think you'll *absolutely love* it,' he says, watching the road, but also seeing the future, it seems.

'I hope so.'

'You will, mate. Don't you think?'

'Yeah.'

'You will.'

We pass the bollard with Gordon Brown's face and turn onto a thinning road. Dad pulls over a few yards before the asphalt fades into a dirt track. 'Can you keep your mobile close by?' I ask, stepping out.

Creepers hold the gates permanently open and climb the lattices against the house wall. I linger beneath the trees and giant grass plants. A pile of wood spills from one of the sheds; an axe stands lodged into an old chopping stump.

I'm only three and a half miles from home. It's only Barrow.

A door I didn't notice opens.

'Ooh, ya bastard!' Boris beckons me in.

My friends are spread out on black sofas in the lounge, in a flushed light from the low sun; seeing this gives me a sensation of being in the nineties.[50]

---

[50] With all the restrictions of childhood, the ever-watching gaze of giant adults, the humiliations they think we forget.

I find a weird organ at the back of the room. Its keys make a tone-less thump under my fingers, until my foot finds a pedal that pumps air into it, like bagpipes. I begin a round of 'Like Spinning Plates', but let it exhale to nothing, conscious that Ben's here, who's an incredible pianist, and that the song is too linked to last autumn, and I feel my old ways grabbing hold of the rope I'm lowering to the past.

In the yard, Boris loads a few cuts of wood into the chiminea, crunches paper up and stuffs it in the bottom, strikes a match with trembling hands. We unfold the iron patio chairs. George gets the axe stuck in the chopping stump, and when nothing else works I use a hammer and chisel to pry the grain open and get it out, whilst Ryan murmurs to Ben something about me "using his Westoby Windows skills", and they both laugh quietly. Sausages crowd a gnarly little grill above the fire.

Emma arrives whilst the others eat, wearing one of my old hoody jackets.

'Check you out,' I say, perching on the stump. 'Do a twirl?'

She totters round on the balls of her feet, then holds her arms out at ten and four.

I smile. 'You do look nice.'

She kneels on the patio, puts her hands on my lap and kisses me. I smell her dad's smoke in her clothes.

'We're all off to the Blow Wells, apparently,' I say.

The track at the end of Boris's road skirts a stubbled crop field, where swarms of tiny midges hang in the sun. I throw chalk stones and tufts of roots as we walk. The Humber Bridge is right there beyond the fields, its tower lights starting to look bright compared to the failing sky. See? As the crow flies, I'm closer to home now than I was at Boris's.

A dry mud path curves through the woods, barely visible in the fuzzy twilight. Dead tree limbs poke out the bogs. A little stream that blocks our way has reduced to sludge. I put my feet on either bank and help Emma jump over, disturbing all the flies. Then over a fallen tree, so decayed that a kick sends up showers of damp chippings.

I take a picture of us all on a wooden bridge.

Emma hesitates when the others keep walking. 'Did you want to take one of me?' she asks.

36

Ben's got one of those strange cassettes with a wire coming out of it: you slot it into your car's stereo and plug the wire into your iPod. As we're circling Millfields roundabout in his tiny car, 'Closer' by Nine Inch Nails comes on. I know it the second that beat starts. I can't hear this. Do I tell him to turn it off? Cover my ears and shout? It's seeping into me. I picture being without God's help. Lost in the panic of imminent humiliation. Begging for his help, his forgiveness. Feeling only his scorn.

But it's not my decision that this is playing.

But it's your decision to allow it to keep *playing.*

I'm sorry. I don't know what to do.

You know what you should *do.*

We pull up at Ben's barely a minute into the track, but it's enough to be marked by it. I drink a few bottles of Budweiser, feeling sick by the end of the first.

37

In Barton youth club, they've cleared the hall out and leather beds are arranged in a big circle. I fill out the form, answer a nurse's questions behind a screen, and get laid down on a bed to give blood. Emma's got an appointment too, but I've made sure to come before she could. I open and close my hand, open and close, lean over to see the sack of blood filling up.

This is a good thing to do.

I fall quiet on the bus into college.

Emma asks what's up, and as always I say 'Nothing' and try to concentrate on breathing exercises.

My first period's a double free. In the Maggy May, I feel a shit churning inside. I can't concentrate on anything else. It's a long, long time until I'm home. Am I getting ill? The volume of chatter and laughter in here is too much. Hundreds of voices, blurring into the images of them all laughing at me, talking about me. It's making me worse.

It shouldn't be this way: I gave blood last night! I did "something amazing", as the adverts said. I spent all night feeling as though God will be looking out for me more than ever for a while, or at least for today.

Wait.

Is giving blood wrong?

Is it... *punishable*?

That can't be true. But the movement in my stomach and the rising dread that I'm going to be ill would suggest maybe it is.

I can't take the noise any longer and go outside, where the sound immediately mutes, from deafening crowds to footsteps on pavement, breeze fluttering in my ears, isolated conversations of those I walk past.

Down the courtyard stairs, past the old smoking shelter and through the outdoor corridor, I take a left into the library. An almost complete silence. A few heads look up from their work as the door shuts behind me with that crinkly sound of its gaskets rubbing together. I head to the reading area and put my iPod in, play the recording I downloaded of Ian McKellen reading *The Rime of the Ancient Mariner* whilst I follow on the print-out.

My attention's thrown whenever I feel the swell in my abdomen.

Should I apologise? Is giving blood a sin? Am I throwing away something God's given to me, as with suicide? Is it because I might be helping someone who shouldn't be helped, and therefore messing with the balance of the world? What religion is it where you're not allowed to give blood or get transfusions?

I thought I'd done something right. Is there no fucking winning? Isn't anything good enough?

Sorry, I shouldn't be mad, as though I understand what's right.

I cycle once again through the questions of sins fitting their punishment. If Boris and Emma gave blood last night, too, why aren't they being punished? They seemed fine this morning. Haven't any of the other millions who've donated blood been punished?

As tiny children sat cross-legged on the bristly purple carpet in primary school, our class was told a story about doing good in the world: the spirit of a dead woman is being judged on whether she's allowed into Heaven, and the only loving deed she ever did in life was give a carrot to a starving tramp. The judging angels produce this very carrot and it kind of pulls her up towards Heaven, like it's attached to a string. Then she screws up. Suddenly noticing a bunch of others clung to her clothing, hitching a ride to Heaven, she tries to swat them all away, which makes her accidentally let go of the carrot.

Is a carrot all it takes?

Will the pint of my blood float before me one day, in zero gravity, for me to grab hold of and be taken up?

In Year Six or Seven, me and Ben spent a morning doing a trick where he waited on the wall on one side of Brigg Road and I hid in a ditch on the other side. When a car came, he shouted 'Now!' and I threw a capillary-like bunch of elderberries up and over the ditch, hopefully hitting the car windscreen. We never gave much thought to how flawed this genius mischief was – that Ben was right there in plain sight. As though, just because the driver didn't see Ben himself throw the berries, they would assume he wasn't involved.

We felt like crooks, but I doubt many drivers gave a shit.

On the way home from berry pelting, Ben told me about an uncle he has who was both a surgeon and something he called an "atheist".

This uncle told Ben that it doesn't matter if you save or fix lives; the only way into Heaven is if you believe in God and Jesus. And since he doesn't, he's off to Hell, according to Christianity. Ben couldn't understand why a shitty person who believes in God can be more holy than a lifesaver who doesn't.

Then in Year Ten, Ben plummeted into a deeply religious phase. He read the Bible and discussed it into the night with groups from the church; he wouldn't hesitate to go on about it in front of our friendship group whilst we gave each other smirking looks; he and Holly had frequent dinners with the local bishop.

One Brazier Night up by his old summerhouse, I brought up what he once told me about his surgeon uncle and asked if he remembered the story about the carrot. He unspooled "famous" interpretations and criticisms of the Bible from throughout the ages, which I couldn't possibly memorise. I just wiped the wet rim of my Newcastle Brown under my top lip, then took another swig. I believed in something back then – I always have.

Ben did a U-turn. With all the intelligence he brought to Christianity, he was bound to start delving into the cracks in its reasoning, the contradictions, until he turned against the whole thing as complete bollocks. It was doomed to play itself out. Nowadays he hauks Bible passages and chucks them into the meat grinder of Logic. He talks about the dark secrets behind Christian holidays and saints. About the Nietzsche books he reads that say "God is dead". He wears a t-shirt with a picture of that guy with long hair and a beret, but I'm not sure what that stands for.

Concentrate.

'The man hath penance done, and penance more will do,' says Ian McKellen in my ears. I turn a few pages to catch up with him.[51] The whole poem's about a sailor's torture for shooting an albatross.

And what if you go to church, pray to and believe in God, do selfless things on a daily basis, but your personality is shit? You finish building wooden schools in the third world, say your prayers, but then laugh at the joke, "If a camera adds ten pounds, do African children even exist?" So long as being horrible doesn't harm anyone, does it not count? I've got to figure this stuff out.

There must be a plan I don't see. I wonder again if this whole world I'm in is a test for me.[52] The reason no one else is governed by

---

[51] Amongst my annotations that crowd the poem I spot words like "divine retribution" and "God's wrath". Like repeatedly meeting a stranger's eye despite myself. What does it mean, that these words stand out from my own handwriting? Are they predictions? A threat? Was I not meant to write such things down, my observations, my notes scribbled in class? Will their meanings turn on me?

[52] But hang on: this thought is close to the lyrics of a Nine Inch Nails song, and possibly inspired by it. "What if everything around you isn't quite as it seems? What if all the world you think you know is an elaborate dream?" Trent Reznor sings. "What if all the world's inside of your head, just creations of your own?" The band has warped my beliefs. I think. *Sorry for letting this happen. It's exactly what you feared. I'll try not to think it.*

this sin-means-punishment system is because they are not real. Or perhaps it's *because* I believe in God that God is punishing me for sinning: he wants to mould me into a better person, and I should be thankful.

Weird Al once rapped about "a local boy" who "kicked me in the butt", going on to say, "I really don't care, in fact I wish him well, 'cause I'll be laughing my head off when he's burning in Hell". Putting aside that it's a piss-taking song, I always thought that's a serious idea. Why bother being mad at horrible people? They'll have a punishment far worse than you could ever serve. Once they die. Once they are dead. That's why I see terrible people in good health. But if judgement is meant to happen when you die, why are there select examples of punishment *in life*? Like with the Ancient Mariner. Like with me.

Did Bitty's dad do something terrible to deserve his daughter's death?

Did *she*?

Glenn Hoddle got axed from managing England football team for the bat-shit claim that disabled people are paying for sins in a previous life. He said Karma trickles through multiple lives. How is it fair, if punishment is meant to make you learn? What amendments can you make when you've no idea what sins you did in your previous life? Google "bad people" and make an educated guess which one of them you were? Scour through criminal records? But the vast majority of sinners aren't documented, aren't prosecuted. How can you combat that, other than praying and trying to be good?

How far back does my window of punishable actions reach? My birth? Childhood? It goes back and back, until it *finds* a sin. So is there any time I should feel so safe as I did last night and this morning? That giving blood made me immune from those towers of past sins that look down on me?

An itch makes itself known in the crook of my arm. I gently rub it, careful not to wake the site the needle entered last night. It's a hot itch. Little bumps are rising around the dot of scab, the skin a bruised yellow.

By the time I leave the library, the feeling in my stomach's gone. I sit down in Literature and send up my thanks to God for forgiving me.

Waiting for the bus on Glover Road, it feels incredible that I've made it through the day. Emma leans back on me and I put my arms around her. Sebastian stands near us and frowns at his iPod, his thumb swirling round the click wheel. Sophia talks loudly to her friends and shows her teeth in a smile.

'Imagine if we'd both known where we'd be now, when we first got together,' Emma says on our way up the hill out of Scunthorpe. 'Like, how many crazy things we know about each other now. How much better we are at stuff.'

'If I'd known in school that I'd be shagging you in the first year of Sixth Form,' I say. Emma laughs and nips me. I laugh too but I'm thinking about something else. 'I'm worried I won't make it to your birthday,' I finally pluck up the courage to say when we're halfway home.

'It'll all be fine. My house hasn't moved. Everyone's going to be there. They've heard so much about you over the last year and two thirds, and they can't wait to meet you. Nanna asks about you every time I see her. Bless her. You have to come. I'll come get you if you don't.'

You've used that joking threat before.

'I will come. You know, I plan to come. I'm just scared of letting you down.'

All the family from down south are coming up. They'll want to know why I always have an excuse not to go down there and see them.

A girl gets up and pulls a window flap open. The fields outside glare yellow with rapeseed blossoms.

'It's like the holiday to Devon and Surrey. I don't know how I'll do it,' I say.

'Sneak me into your suitcase. I'll make sure you're alright.'

38

Grand Theft Auto IV comes out. I watch the video reviews online. I know from the past the kind of things you can do in *GTA* games. Beat up, gun down or run over pedestrians. Sleep with hookers, then kill them so you don't have to pay. Follow a campaign where you work for crime organisations. The reviewers talk about the story's dark tone, the no-win decisions you must make as a player. And that it's one of the best games ever. I buy it, and when it comes, leave it in the cellophane wrapper and store it in a drawer. I'll play it when I turn eighteen.

I worry that I'll be punished just for buying it. For wanting it. For having it in that drawer. Emitting its unholy corruption, like when the box in *Raiders of the Lost Ark* kills the rats surrounding it in the cargo hold.

I've played 18s all my life. I find the case for *Call of Duty*: it's 16+, so that's okay. I dig out *Gears of War* and *Bioshock*: both 18s. Was I punished around the times of playing them? Come to think of it: yes. I was getting worse in the autumn of 2006, when I'd play *Gears of War*, often with Jordan or Emma. Were *they* punished? And *Bioshock* was in the following autumn, when I wasn't managing college at all. Yet, I've also played it this spring, and been mostly fine. What pattern am I missing?

I bury *GTA* deeper into the drawer, beneath the old cards I never gave Dad, so I don't have to see it. And I fight the urge to just throw it away.

39

Me and Jordan pull up an old plum tree stump at my grand-parents'. The last tree left of what was once a little orchard, where the ground was soft under strange hair-like grass; a thick, sweet smell hung in the air; wasps whipped around and landed in the burrows they'd made in the cooking apples and plums. I doubt Jordan's old enough to remember.

It's a hot day. Mum, Grandma and Granddad are in the old conservatory, occasionally watching with a nod and smile as we hoik roots out the ground. The bruise around my needle hole has darkened to a shade of purple. My arm's stiffened up like a sprain and it's been a week since I could train biceps. Holding a spade like a barbell, I look down and study whether my muscles have shrunk.

Dad stands over the barbeque, his face its familiar shade of red after a few glasses of wine. He holds his palm above the grate, shakes it and remarks that the coals are ready. Picks up the pack of raw chicken wings and starts laying them onto the heat. Puts the empty pack on Bentley's hutch, wipes his fingers on his jeans whilst taking a sip of wine. Bentley runs around his feet.

A gust of wind makes the smoke whirl around the garden.

I'll be eighteen in a month.

I go inside and dial the number for a driving instructor. A guy with a Yorkshire accent answers. He's free next week.[53]

'Erm, okay,' I say, too slow to invent a reason to put it off.

It's better this way, maybe. Less time to worry.

---

[53] That soon? But I was digging the garden at Grandma's. I had to wash my hands with their soap. There was old bird shit on the stump we pulled up. Moss. Shreds of bark coming off in my hands. Me and Emma had sex last night, and I put my trousers on later without washing my hands first because it seemed rude to immediately wash her (and myself) off me. A man with a gigantic Toys "R" Us bag sat next to me on the bus the other day. Some rain water landed on my tear duct when I looked up to the sky. All the particles that transfer from Emma's carpet onto my socks, and then I put my feet up on the sill at home before remembering I need to take them off, and then I saw Mum touch the sill to steady herself whilst drawing the curtains, and then she might have prepared food before washing her hands. When I showered earlier today, the towel I used may have collected residual particles of grass from cutting Grandma's lawn. I might forget to sneak it into the wash basket next time Mum's not around, and end up using it again, wiping my face with it. Can an illness from these things hibernate for a week? Awaken in the confines of a learner car where me and the instructor sit so close? I've heard he nearly always takes you to Scunthorpe, or even *Cleethorpes*.

After putting the phone down I wash my hands.[54] Dry my hands on kitchen roll whilst asking Mum if she ever cleans the phone.

The cuts on my knuckles sting long after they're dry.

40

Foxy's got a skinhead, big teeth, a big shout. He probably doesn't remember, but when I was in reception year of primary school and he was in year six, he stole one of my Pogs and refused to admit it to the dinner lady when I grassed him up. I knew it was him. I wanted to cry. He's an amateur boxer now, always messing up his haymaking shoulder. We sometimes spot each other at the gym. Most of his stories are about fights he was in at the weekend. A broken jaw here, teeth falling across the pavement there, cutting down a side street when the sirens approach. The stories end with his cackling laugh, like scrunching a pack of crisps in your hands. I ask him to teach me to box. After our workouts we shut ourselves in the studio room and he corrects my stance, where my fists should float in front of me, how to twist my elbow into a punch.

I've got the gloves on; he holds up the pads and shouts at me whilst I twat his hands. He smacks me when I forget my guard. I go until my calves are on fire, my shoulders fuzzy and weak.

'Ten more seconds. Fucking go for it now. Let's fucking go,' he booms.

I shout through my teeth and give it everything.

'Alright, alright. Jesus I'm in the fucking corner.'

---

[54] I've seen Dad answer the phone at the dinner table when I know his hands aren't clean. I've seen him re-arrange his junk and pick the phone up minutes later. And think of all the *breath* that's floated into the transmitter, with us all talking into it for all these years. Warm, wet breath. After eating who knows what. Talking on the phone when we have a cold, even a sickness bug. And the waxy ears the receiver has rested against. I should shower again.

He cackles, tears the velcro from his wrists with his teeth[55] and throws the pads away.

I pull my hands out the boxing gloves; they absolutely stink.

If Foxy's not around, I wrap up my wrists and hit the punch bag for a while. Never in gloves: I like how it only takes eight or nine punches for the skin to start pulling off my knuckles in thick white flaps, leaving raw patches. I keep punching, and even if I'm scared an infection will pass from the bag's dirty leather to my exposed wounds, I enjoy the pain. *Fuck you, fuck you*, I think with each hit, and the blue leather gets darker and darker.

41

It's time. You can do this.

Dear God, please let me be alright today. If I need to be ill, please let it be when I get home, not whilst I'm at Emma's. Please let me be okay. Even if I don't deserve it, then for Emma's sake. She's the nicest person in the world, and this is her day. She deserves it to go well. Don't let me be the one to ruin it. She deserves the best day. Amen.

'Chris, we're going,' Mum shouts up the stairs.

I check my reflection in James's old surfboard mirror and hurry downstairs, wriggle my feet into my shoes and wait in the car. The flurry of images goes on. I think of escapes and hiding places at the party. Calculate hours until nightfall. Hours until it'd be acceptable to leave. My parents and Jordan are coming, too. Having the car there's an advantage, but they won't stay late. I look down at my thumbnails and consider talking to God again. Have I prayed enough? I prayed last night. And at the gym this morning, pressing dumbbells above my head and punching blood into the bag.

It's overcast. There's a marquee set up in Emma's garden, and her dad has attached big sheets of blue tarpaulin from the wall to the fence, extending the shelter. Balloons, banners, weird sequin things,

---

[55] Insane.

hang from its ceiling. Her family's everywhere, all with thick London accents. I get asked whether I support Arsenal or Chelsea by a bickering pair of uncles. Jordan hits it off with a younger cousin. Emma's grandma asks me what I'm going to be. The small talk between mine and Emma's parents is predictably painful. I dream of it being time to go home, so many hours from now. A playlist Emma made beside me one afternoon on the sofa now booms through her dad's stereo, which he's got rigged up under the tarpaulin. Text after text comes through off our friends, cancelling on Emma. I get increasingly mad, especially with people like Ben, whose excuse is ridiculous and I know he could easily have come. I also get worried that fewer friends here will make it all the worse if I leave. Emma drops her hands to her sides and says 'Fuck's sake' when another text comes through. She holds up the phone to me: it's from Holly. We're in the kitchen, by the big spread of party food on the table.

'It's ridiculous,' I say, and bundle her up in a hug.

'I'm watching you!' Emma's grandma says through the bannisters.

She and Emma laugh; I manage a smile and exhale.

Back outside, the tarpaulin casts a shade of blue on us all. Emma sips her Malibu and lemonade, holding the straw with her free hand and occasionally tapping the bed of the glass with it. She wears a massive 18th badge. 'Aren't you having a beer?' she asks.

'Later on, yeah.' Though I wish I didn't have to.

My family leaves by dinner time, and I carry on doing what I always do at these kind of parties: make slow laps between the house and marquee, try to look occupied, watch the clock, pretend I'm not out of place with no one to talk to. I'm thankful whenever a member of Emma's family says, 'It's Chris, right?' and introduces themselves.

Emma's summoned to open the presents that have collected by the stereo. Her relatives form a circle around her and tame jokes float in from the comedians amongst them. Emma's mum emerges with a lit cake and we all sing.

I'm at the back of the crowd, on my toes to see Emma. But I daren't push through and step into the limelight. These people have more of a right to be here than me: they've known her since she was born. I keep hoping she'll look for me in the crowd and invite me up to be next to her. It's like she doesn't know how hard it was to come here.

Her dad, pretty drunk by now, puts his arm around her and tells her to make a speech.

'Thank you all for coming,' is all she manages before her head shrinks into her shoulders and her cheeks burn. The family laughs and goes '*aww*'.

In the evening a few friends arrive and get drinking in the darkest quarter of the marquee. I manage a beer and feel pangs of excitement that it's nearly an acceptable time to go home. At eleven I text Dad to come get me.

Emma's hurt that I'm going. Family members catch wind and say, 'You're *going*? Come on!'

'I've got to go,' is all I can think to say, fake laughing, in a "believe me, I wish I didn't have to leave" kind of way.

Is it so outrageous? It's been eight hours!

Emma clings onto me in the hallway. It's the most I've seen of her today. Emma's dad is smoking out the front with his brother.

'Is that your dad's car?' he asks.

'Yeah, I'm heading home.'

He blocks the doorway. 'You don't have to go, mate. You can stay here if you want.'

Between each offer is an awkward pause where I smile and do the "sadly, I can't" half-shrug, not knowing where to look. 'Walk like an Egyptian' plays in the garden.

'What do you reckon? You can stay if you want.'

'He needs to go, Dad.'

'Aw, you should stay. Emma wants you to.' He pushes himself off the doorjamb. 'Have a good one, mate. We'll see you next week, yeah?'

'Definitely. See you soon. Thanks a lot.'

'Thanks for coming,' Emma says at the gate. 'Love you.'

She kisses me. I lick my lips and taste pineapple.

* * *

Shit, I haven't said thank you!

I jolt awake from the fringe of a dream, like the sensation of falling.

Dear God, sorry I've only just remembered to pray. You've watched over me and I completely forgot to tell you I'm thankful, like I promised I would. Sorry. There's no excuse. I was caught up in the party and trying to be okay. Thank you for keeping me safe. Thank you. Thank you. Please let Emma be happy and having a great time if she's still awake there.

When I get to the end of the prayer, I let myself slip away. I dream that we're returning to Florida. A dream that comes every month or so: either we're *in* Florida and I'm counting the days until we come home again, or, like tonight, I'm trapped in the run-up to going there, convinced that there's only a few days left until we're on that plane, and a two week stretch of heat and fear waits ahead.

42

'I don't know how I can manage Devon.'

Mum's curling her eyelashes. She goes a little rigid. 'You've managed college so far this year,' she says. 'What's the difference in going on a holiday?'

I'm knelt on the floor, my arms folded on my parents' bed.

'Going to Scunthorpe's a little different to going seven or eight hours to Devon, and then whatever it is from there to Surrey.'

'We'll be in your dad's car. There'll be plenty of service stations.'

As she says that, my head blossoms with scenes of me begging us to hurry up to the services. Squeezed in the back of the car with my brothers. Sick and desperate.

'That – that doesn't matter.'

'You've been doing so well.'

'It will be too much, though. I'm worried that if it goes terribly then it'll knock me back, even.'

She swings round with a frown and her bottom lip turned down, then turns back to the dressing table mirror and puts her eyelash curler in the little bag of ablutions.

'Well you know how James was having similar problems before he went to Spain a couple of years ago. Now look how he's doing. This could be your Spain.'

'It's not the same.'

At least I've laid the foundations. It won't be as big a shock when I say flat-out that I can't go.

43

Revision steps up another gear. My bedroom has assessment objectives blu-tacked to the wall. I spend the sunny days sheltered in the college library memorising notes, making them smaller and smaller, into bullet points I can then expand into sections of essays. Re-reading Lit's primary texts over and over.

Me and Emma cross the main road and lie on the sports field. The ice cream paedophile's back, with a queue of students stemming from his van. I attempt to organise my words and tell Emma what bothered me about her party. She nods along and plucks at the grass.

'Sorry. I was trying to keep everyone entertained. All my family. You could've just stuck with me. I would've loved that. It's all I wanted.'

A forty-eight-hour grudge melts away. What the hell's wrong with me?

'I didn't mean it should've been more about me. No way. I just felt like I'd put all that effort into coming – it was so fucking hard – and it barely mattered that I was there in the end.'

'It *did* matter. I had to go upstairs and cry for a while when you left. Because everyone was asking where you were and why you'd left. It's the first time I finally got to show you off to my family and prove you're not, you know, make believe, and you left barely halfway through the party.'

'It was eleven o'clock.'

'And it went on until nearly three.'

'I didn't realise it was so important I stayed.'

A magpie lands near us, nips a discarded pastry, hops a few feet forward and takes off again. Most of its catch breaks apart and drops to the grass. I salute to it whilst Emma's looking down, tip my head back and let the sun warm my closed eyelids.

'I should've stayed longer,' I say. 'It was just very hard.'

But even as I say it, I wonder if I'm lying. It was terrifying to go, after weeks of worrying, making sure I was perfectly sterile and perfectly innocent, but an hour or so in, if that, was the fear really there? Did I leave because it was hard, or was I just desperate to reach the finish line? For the *hard thing* to be done and dusted. Achieved. I certainly didn't want to sleep over. But Dad probably would've picked me up later, considering it was Emma's eighteenth. I could've walked home; it would only have taken an hour and a half. Have I lied? *Sorry, Lord. I don't know. I could have tried harder. I prayed for Emma's happiness but I was the one who stopped it.*

'Dad got so drunk,' Emma says.

'Yeah?'

'He ended up throwing up in the bath. Him and my uncle are like kids again whenever they get together. It was so funny.' She laughs.

I smile.[56]

We go for a walk through the woods that go down the hill after the tennis courts. The paths are dry and dusty. Bikers have carved tall ramps into the steep slopes. I sit on my heel and slide down one, like we used to at Death Hill, into a bowl where the ramps meet.

---

[56] Is Emma positive it's the alcohol that made him throw up? It might have been something else. A sickness bug. It's plausible. What if Emma's carrying it now? Or even if it was the booze, vomit itself must be riddled with bacteria. What if Emma came into contact with it and now it's passed onto me?

There are scorched fire pits, booze bottles and tins, newspapers and ruined porn mags, a syringe.

'Come on!' Emma shouts from above. 'I'm not going down there.'

I scramble back up the slope. There's dog shit everywhere. Dark and dry or wet like caramel. Clustered with flies that disperse if you get too close. Think of all the places the flies go after eating shit. Landing on us humans, our food; we shake them off and continue eating.

Emma puts her arms through my jacket and kisses me. We hug at the top of a slope for a while. Making up. I feel an inappropriate boner coming on and stealthily turn my pelvis away. But she notices and rubs her palms up and down it, over my jeans. I reach down her back, under her trousers and feel her French knickers tight against her arse.

'If only we could do it,' Emma says.

'E-Block toilets?' I laugh. 'Or what if we...' I take her hand and we go a few yards down the path, cut into the trees. We come across a tiny clearing. I look at Emma and tilt my head.

She kisses me again. We clutch at each other, suck air in, soak each other in. I undo her trouser buttons.

'Chris,' she says.

'We'll be fine.'

She whispers a laugh.

I pull her trousers down and guide her knees to the ground. Get my emergency condom out the bottom of my bag. We both sigh when I push inside her. We're looking about through the bushes and trees. It's so intense, I want to come straight away. Then I spot a couple and their dog walking up the path. I thought we were deeper into the trees than this!

'Fuck, there's people,' I say.

'Quick then!'

I pump as fast as I can, grab her hips and come. Emma risks a little moan, but I regret she didn't get chance to orgasm.

We jump to our feet, hoist our trousers up and grab our bags. My boxers feel slimy. I fling the condom behind me and act casual, stepping back onto the path just as the couple come past. Their brown Labrador comes to look up at us and wags its big tail.

Once they've passed, I pull Emma into another kiss. She has a big rosy smile.

'You're so flushed,' I laugh. 'Oh no, am I too?'

'Very.' She rubs my sides under my t-shirt, then takes my hand.[57] We head back to college. 'I'm pretty sure they knew what we were up to.'

'The dog certainly knew something.'

44

In the final Art assessment I paint a series of bright colour plumes, tiled unevenly together like a zoomed-in mosaic. For the analysis I write how different the style is to last year's meticulous biro drawings, and that it has a personal significance to me. Last year I was shrunk, my head down, scratching tiny details together to distract myself. I'm not so confined anymore: the spacious paintings represent literal distances I can cross, a relaxed mindset. As I write these things, it's like I'm closing a chapter. I'm out the other side of whatever kept me in Barton, at home. The story's done.

---

[57] Must, must wash my hands once we're back in college. The dirtiness clings like treacle on my skin. I've touched my bag strap with *sex juice* hands! And it's not only that. There's the grass I touched back on the field, a branch I impulsively grabbed here in the woods, and a reeling list of other bad surfaces since I left home this morning. But the sinks in college will have far more germs. So do I not wash my hands? I can't not wash them. I don't know. Literature is in an hour – I can't sit there and not touch my pencil case or notebook. People will ask questions. Will Emma wash hers? Surely. Shall I avoid letting her touch me for the rest of the day, to be safe? Keep an eye on what parts of herself she touches with those hands: brushing her hair back, rubbing an eye, letting her hands fall by her sides? I can't do that to her. But the exams are coming.

45

I'm on my laptop at home, tuning the recent pictures I've taken: Emma's party, close-ups of leaves, bark, the fluffy cobwebs that grow in the scars of old branches, tiny pink stems stretching from moss patches on a wall on Glover Road, a sudden mist we got one night.

Then it occurs to me: is Photoshop bad, since I got it illegally from the college technician? Is this why some residual punishments have leaked through?

My finger recoils from the touchpad.

There's no victim. Adobe, who make Photoshop, is a multimillion-dollar company. What difference does me using a copy make?

Being a big company doesn't mean there aren't "little" people working there, trying to get by. Photoshop sales pay their wages. What if this pirate copy knocks Adobe over a financial tipping point, and in some lowest-rung office, a guy has to be let go?

What if no one in Adobe ever notices, but Leggott gets onto the technician's case for handing these copies out, and he gets fired?

Down swoops a thought: *You should give whatever money it would've cost to charity.*

I don't have that much money.

Then give away what you do *have.*

My finger hovers above the touchpad.

I shut the laptop.

46

I slide a twenty-kilogram plate on either side of the heavy bar, pick it off the floor and bicep curl it. My arms only get halfway up, but it gets a screaming pump going.

'You've been having your Weetabix,' remarks the guy who steps outside the gym to smoke a few times per workout.

'Cheers.' I put the barbell down, immediately grab the dumb-bells beside my feet.

I talk to a massive, spherical ex-firefighter. He's got constantly bulging eyes, like everything I say comes as the shock of his life. 'I'm a teetotaler, me,' he declares. 'I don't go out and get smashed. Me and the Mrs like to stay in and watch films, you know? Put something nice on.' Then he lies back and presses some fifties like they're sugar bags.

'I'm sick whenever I drink. I barely have enough to feel anything, then later on I'll feel terrible,' I say when he sits back up.

'Where is it you're going, anyway?'

'Either Huddersfield or Nottingham Trent.'

'It's good that you're off. Get out of this place. There's nowt here for you to make of yourself. Then in a few years' time you'll be driving around in an M3 and I'll be in my little banger, still.'

'I doubt it.' I smile.

'Just make sure you remember us when you're rich.' He knees the weights up to his chest and lies back for another set.

Later on in the changing rooms he's at the sink, cracking eggs into his protein shaker. 'I got a bit of shell off that one.'

Dean's leant by the microwave with his arms folded, watching. 'You drink the yolks, too?'

'Yeah, there's no use trying to keep them out.'

He lets the fourth egg drool into the shaker, then adds a scoop of chocolate protein powder, and another. He pulls a small bottle of milk from his sports bag and pours it in.

'I lost me lid for this so I've brought a fork for stirring.' He stirs with his fork and the whole thing turns a vile dark brown with swirling streaks of yolk.

'The fucking lumps,' Dean says, his grin broadening. 'Are you going to drink that?'

'I've had worse in my mouth.'

'Eugh. Poo?'

'Yeah,' the fireman says between gulps, wet brown on his smiling lips, his eyes bulging.

Another workout session, Foxy and his mate are there. Foxy's on about a student he's been banging.

'Put your thumb up her arse and bowl her out the door, mate,' he says. 'They love it.'

Bowl her out the door?

'Fucking students, though. Seriously, like. The student nights round Hull. I don't care who I fucking take back. You know? Didn't you say you're off to uni?'

'Yeah,' I say, grinning but uncomfortable.

'Fucking hell. Fucking buff fucker like you. Your balls won't be dry for one fucking minute. Girls will be fucking gushing.' He gets a foot up on one of the benches and wriggles his fingers away from his crotch. Laughs his massive cackle. Smacks his mate on the chest with the back of his hand.

That aching tension you feel in your cheek muscles, that you only notice when your smile isn't real.

I laugh along whilst saying sorry to God.

47

The front door unlocks; I look up from my work at the kitchen table.

Nanna comes in, wearing her white cardigan and baby blue trousers.

'Aww. I really thought you'd be going this time.'

'I know.'

'When did they go?'

'About...' I lean to see the oven clock '...twenty minutes ago.'

Yes, I paced room to room. Got dressed like I was going with them, then sat on my bed and thought, *I can't*. Shook the thought off and put texturising gum in my hair. Ready to roll. Wondered whether I was going to be ill. Pictured illness roiling on the motorways, in the city I've never seen. I sat back down at my desk. Stared at the assessment objectives stuck to my wall.

'We're probably going to pick up James, get a bite to eat somewhere, maybe go back to his for a cuppa. That's all,' Mum said here in the kitchen, tying up the bin bag.

I was leant on the corner of the table.

'We won't even be that long. Hour, hour and a half there. Couple hours in town. James will be over the moon if you came. Hey?' Dad said. Another massive underestimation. I knew it wouldn't be until this evening that they'll be home.

Their encouragement only weighed me down: I was going to disappoint them.

'I should probably revise.'

As they left I yearned to go with them so much, like I was stretching into two; part of me was heading out there and getting in the car. Every second was another opportunity to think *fuck it*, jump up and follow them. I sat here hesitating. Holding my forehead, pressing my feet into the floor alternately, as though running. But as the door shut and locked, and the car's engine faded down the street, that stretching tether snapped. I'm left with the decision I made. Missing James's birthday.

'Come and see this,' Nanna says now.

I squeeze from behind the table. Nanna sits a white carrier bag on the counter and opens it. There's a big log-shaped cut of pork, its pale fat squeezing between the red string lattice.

The smell of Nanna's talcum powder strays up my nose.

'Fiver. That's all I paid.'

She looks at me, holding open the bag, so I do an impressed nod.

48

The exams are close. In the middle of walking down to the gym, cuddling Emma on her sofa, trying to study, I slip into long daydreams of humiliation, the struggle and excruciating time it takes to get home, or how I might excuse myself from the exam room, my insides squeezing sick and shit from me. I plan escapes, hiding places, the routes and times to both. But it's possible I'm not thinking about them as much as last year. Because behind the exams, dwarfing them, is Devon, in all its concrete impossibility. There's nothing after it.

49

I still own that old *Of Mice and Men* book our class was each given in Year Eleven to study and return. Choosing to steal it: another offence I haven't fixed. I should ask Jordan if he'll take it with him to school on Monday and give it to Mr. Scarason with my apologies for accidentally keeping it. Or deliver it myself and explain. And what about the sweets I used to steal from the newsagent's in Year Seven? Nearly every day to and from school I'd hide my hand up my coat sleeve, then sort of scan my sleeve over the shelves of Triple Flip Pops and penny sweets. My hidden fingers would stroke over the goods whilst I looked at the shopkeeper, then claw up a little handful and retract into the sleeve again, before nonchalantly dropping the haul into my pocket, like an elephant's trunk sucking up peanuts. I thought it was ingenious, until I heard the shopkeeper was asking people what my name was. The newsagent's has changed hands a couple of times since then. Should I go back there and pay, or track down whoever owned it at the time?

50

'How long have you had it in there?' James looks excited but confused when I pull *Grand Theft Auto* out the drawer and pickle off the cellophane with a fingernail. God, it feels thrilling. Sacrilege. So wrong but so right. I repeat to myself, *I'm eighteen now. This is okay. I'm eighteen now. It's my choice.* But have I passed into my eighteenth, officially? Today's my birthday, but what if I wasn't born until the afternoon, so technically I'm still underage?

We got up early this morning so I could open the presents from my family before work and school. James is home for a few days, and college lessons have finished, so we get the morning together.

I get a long, gleeful *Happy birthday* text from Emma. And soon after, *Im ready with all your prezzys, can I come round?xxxxxx*

Fuck's sake, I think, shutting my phone, worried and disappointed that the rest of the day will be spent with her. It feels wrong to say no. Or even suggest meeting later on. She's probably sat by her front door waiting for the signal.

Sure xxx I write. Can't I relax on my birthday? The game hasn't even finished installing.

The little knock at the front door.

I head downstairs and see bright balloons through the wobbly glass.

'Happy birthday!' Emma cheeps, her arms full with cards, presents, the balloon ribbons.

'Oh my God,' I say with a beaming laugh, my heart sinking.

Emma's here, in the **morning**. She will want to stay all day.

But I'm touched, and guilty. I upset her on her birthday and she's still done this. My birthday is a happy event to her; it makes my smile real, despite everything.

* * *

I try to organise a party for the coming Saturday. But only a few of the texts I get back say they are free. Then on Saturday the run of sunshine ends and it mizzles all morning. More friends drop out and I call the whole thing off.

Everyone will be at Charlie's Bar, I know it. It's where they meet now.

Emma asks if she can come over: *I can cheer u up!xxx*

I'm miles from in the mood to see her but give in eventually. We lie on my bed and talk softly, listen to the rain pick up for a while. I prop my pillow up and turn on *Grand Theft Auto*; feelings of guilt and danger dangle from it. Emma describes her dad's copy of *Doom* she would play as a child, then she seems to fall asleep.

The people you shoot in *Grand Theft Auto* don't die straight away. They crumple, involuntarily shooting their gun all over the place on their way down to a breathing heap on the ground. Some try and get back to their feet, look for their weapon, stumbling like they're drunk. But most clutch the part of them the bullet got, and slowly bleed to death. I fill them with more bullets to end their pain. People who you steal from cling to their car desperately as you drive away in it.

I turn off the game and shuffle closer to Emma. Stroke her hair away and kiss the warm bit of forehead. Her body's roasting.

51

The last days leading to the exams are pure. Every possible sin is a landmine I step around. I see some from a mile away[58], some

---

[58] Not to play *Grand Theft Auto* or *Bioshock*. Not to use mounted turrets or weapons that involve fire on *Call of Duty* or *Uncharted*. Not to use God's name in vain: always keep that in mind in case I suddenly stub a toe or become angry. As well as the obvious songs I can't listen to, there are certain CDs I got for my birthday to add. Don't listen to *Yankee Hotel Foxtrot* by Wilco (as there's a song called 'Jesus, etc.'), *Street Horrrsing* by Fuck Buttons (because of their abrasive sound and name, and the screaming where I can't hear what he says but it seems to involve the word "angels"), *Sea Change* by Beck (because he's into Scientology, apparently). I can't risk 'Yeah (Crass Version)' by LCD Soundsystem (maybe because of the "crass" in the name or because one line sounds like he says "the shit's got to run"), 'Paris is Born' by Laurent Pepper (not sure why), *Illinoise* by Sufjan Stevens (which references God in good ways, but sometimes not, such as, "We lift our hands and pray over your body but nothing ever happens", or "And He takes, and He takes, and He takes"), *The Moon and Antarctica* by Modest Mouse (numerous unfavourable God references), the *There Will Be Blood* soundtrack by Jonny Greenwood (for the cross on the front cover). I try not to remember Nine Inch Nails lyrics: when the song 'Reptile' is stuck in my head, and nothing can stop it replaying, I try to replace the syllables of the line "Angels bleed from the tainted touch of my caress" with "No, no, no, no, no, no no no no no no no". If any memory of a porn video comes to mind I swat it away. I'm careful of what my family's got on TV at night, poised to leave the room if anything anti-God comes on.

in the last moment.[59] Every spare minute between revision sessions, I ask myself if there's anything I must apologise to God for.

The days are also clean.[60] My hands are raw pink after vigorous washes. Saturated skin loose over the knuckles. Then they parch, crinkle and crack like crepe paper. Old man's hands. I change clothes multiple times a day. A change of jeans[61] might lead me to wonder what other clothes I'm wearing that the jeans have touched, so I change my t-shirt, my underwear. Tell off anyone who sits on my

---

[59] Emma's dad talks about God one night. 'I'd have some questions for him if ever we met,' he says menacingly from his chair below the child's frog painting. And I'm in a knot whether to nod along to him to be polite or tell him off/walk out. When a friend makes a crude joke, I try to land between pretending to laugh but not enough to seem like I'm in on the joke or agree with its material. I might be scrolling though iTunes and then become distracted by work, only to look up at my laptop later and see the mouse cursor is hovering too close to Nine Inch Nails. For some reason I can't delete the music completely.

[60] Wash hands after touching the fridge, cupboards, door handles, doors, my shoes (which I try to carry around with my feet), taps (which I try to turn off with my wrist, then avoid touching my wrist with the opposite hand), furniture, any plant, a person, certain areas of my own clothes, foods (since my foody fingers will then touch something else, and that essence of food will spoil, waiting to be touched again and transferred into my mouth), tissue, bins, the inside or out of my parents' cars, certain game cases, light switches and the dangly cord for the bathroom extractor fan. Do as much with my feet and elbows as possible. Avoid the yellow highlighter Boris put in his mouth, and everything related to it. Wash hands after use of all papers and stationery from my backpack just in case, because of the times I touched these things after washing my hands at a toilet in college, after me and Emma did it in the woods, or the times someone else borrowed a pen. Stay away from Grandma's. Don't touch the yellowed newspaper in my room stuffed beside the drawers that might release the past like spores. Careful of the places on the carpet and bed where me and Emma have done stuff, the bottom of the bed where my feet go, where unwashed clothes have landed on the floor and where the mite lotion might have rubbed off.

[61] After walking behind the hoover, for example, and feeling its hot air (which certainly carries dust from the floor, and possibly even *old* dust from inside the machine, picked up years ago, maybe at a time when someone with a sickness bug walked on the patch of floor this old dust was picked up from, and became stuck in the machine in a place that can't be reached when the container's emptied, but today lifts free) caress my leg.

bed. I think about dust, germs, human illness, transferring through the innumerable touches that make a network, a web. I think about the dog shit in the woods with the flies clustered on it. Everything I've done over the last week that might have planted the seeds of illness.

I would watch *Saving Private Ryan* again to make my nerves seem ridiculous, but it doesn't feel right: a film that has made money portraying the suffering of all those people. Not to mention its references to God, like that guy who quotes the Bible whilst aiming sniper shots. Watching that might have been one of the problems keeping me in the mire of punishments.

Instead, I boil the kettle and pour scalding water over the head of my toothbrush, to make sure any germs between those bristles are dead. I take the new Parker pen my parents got me for my birthday out its case and carefully wrap masking tape round it. This stops my hand slipping down it when I sweat.[62]

It feels wrong replacing the old pen: an identical Parker found in the depths of an odds-and-sods drawer at the end of last winter. It's Mum's from when she was a twenty-something ward nurse, her maiden name inscribed on it, spelled wrong: *Sister Worden.* Putting it in my pencil case coincided quite perfectly with the beginning of my recovery. The pen's been with me whilst I've slowly attended more and more lessons, in my hands making notes and drawing doodles down the margin as I've slowly felt more comfortable. It's a betrayal to get rid of it. What if, in some way I don't understand, this pen is one of the reasons I'm better now, and I'm replacing it?

The new pen was a gift. It will look after me.

What the fuck am I talking about?!

Sorry. It's not stupid.

---

[62] But masking tape absorbs the hand's sweat and grease. I've seen it darken in time with the old pen.

52

Dear God, thank you so much for taking care of me this term. Everything's gotten better and better. It means the absolute world to me. I can feel your protection when I'm away and frightened. It's what gives me strength. I know you're there with me. If there's anything I can do to repay you, please send a sign. Please let me know, and I'll do it. Please look over me today, and in the other exams. This is what everything's built up to. I know you'll protect me. If I deserve it. If I've done anything wrong, please forgive me. I don't mean to. I don't mean to offend you. Sorry. If now's the time I have to be punished, I understand, but I hope you can forgive me. Amen. And look over Emma. Please. And my family. My brothers. My parents, who work so hard. Please keep them all safe and happy. I know you will. Thank you. Amen.

Submerged in prayer, the world is quieter. My attention returns here, the aisle of a rammed-full bus where I'm stood, but I keep my eyes shut a moment longer.

The rattling metal and roaring engine. The rabble of the passengers, their screams and stabbing laughter. The blustering air through the windows. The metal bar my hand grips.[63] My body tipping this way and that. It feels like we're in Winterton.

We pull into a stop in the marketplace. I open my eyes. Two more students step on, holding their bus cards out like crosses to a vampire. A frayed young mother seesaws a pram up with one hand and hoists a toddler boy with the other. A yellowed dog follows, the warm morning already making its little tongue dip up and down from its mouth.

'Good morning!' the bus driver calls.

---

[63] The germs practically tangible under my palm. Like when I used to fish and would clutch a handful of maggots from the tub and they squirmed inside my fist to get free, muscling between my fingers.

Revision I've bludgeoned myself with comes out the end of my new Parker. It's like finally having a piss after waiting all day.

On the ride home, I'm determining whether I can celebrate by playing *Grand Theft Auto* for an hour before I carry on revising for the next exam, the day after tomorrow. Probably not worth risking punishment.

I scroll through my iPod for something to listen to. I almost play *Odelay* by Beck – so what if he's a Scientologist? – but it opens with a track called 'Devil's Haircut'. That's the deal-breaker.

After the second exam, I wait outside the gates for my driving instructor's red Citroen: I'm finally one of those kids you see being picked up from college for a driving lesson.

Before the third exam, I go to the library again. I tell myself it's to do some last-minute cramming. But really, I just find the library comforting.

When the last exam ends, I roll the end of my Parker on the paper to clean the deposit of ink it collects on the ballpoint, click the top and listen to the invigilator tell us how to leave the hall in an orderly fashion.

That's it. It's fucking over.

Mum rings me.

'Ah, now then. How did it go?'

'It was only that General Studies exam today. Which might as well have just said, "What do you think about *stuff*?"'

'Well it's done, now. I'm just in Tesco, and remembered you finished at three. Do you want a lift back? I can pick you up if you want.'

'Sure,' I say.

Hanging up, I'm almost disappointed not to be taking the bus home one more time. I wonder whether to ring back and tell her not to come, just for the sake of feeling closure.

At home, I make a cup of tea and go upstairs to my room. Turn on the PS3 and sit back, holding the drink to my chest even though it's a warm day.

Thank you, I say, my eyes looking up beyond the ceiling.

Could it be the world's falling into place?

53

I take my jeans and t-shirt off, then carefully lay them on the wicker chair in the corner of my room. Grab a fresh towel from the airing cupboard and close the bathroom door behind me. Use my feet to take each sock off, lift the lid off the wash basket and lift my foot up to drop them in, toppling off balance for a moment in this weird yoga pose.

Emma's knock sounds downstairs as I'm scrubbing my hair dry in my room. The front door gets unlocked and I shout for Emma to come up. I like to appear busy when she arrives; it's easier to cope with than the formality of me opening the door.

We walk down Ferriby Road, alongside another hedge I used to pluck a leaf from without fail.

Charlie's Bar is loud and bright. Heads turn as we come in and their stares hold. Blokes eye Emma, then me. Like meat, like shit. They don't move when I try to squeeze round them, saying, '–scuse me.' The bartender eventually breaks free of her view of the TV screen, comes over and looks at me.

'Glass of coke, please, and a Malibu and lemonade.'

The guy right beside us turns his stool to face me, though I can't be sure it's me he is staring at because I don't really want to look.

Our group's in the beer garden, around a big wooden table, with a few people I don't know. It's a scratty little area, but the evening sun is warm out here. It turns the white paving slabs a peach colour. The table's full. Ciders and ice cubes, beers and lagers, mixers, little stacks of empty glasses that Wykes adds to after letting the last dregs of his cider slide into his mouth. Their laughter's louder than usual. I wish I wasn't here.

I don't know how to join the table; there's something impenetrable about it. Me and Emma perch on a neighbouring bench and I put a big smile on, to seem like I'm having fun, like them.

Ant leans back on his seat to see me. 'What you drinking?'

'Just this,' I say, holding up my coke.

'Aw, no,' he laughs. 'Aren't you drinking?'

Most of the table's turned to look at us. One of the girls asks Emma if she's alright.

'Just tired,' Emma says, which is *always* her answer.

'Tired from riding my long, *hard* cock,' Ant butts in. The whole group blows up in laughter, tipping back and saying 'Oooh!' and 'You can't say that', looking to me for my reaction.

I laugh behind my smile and feel a coil of anger heating up. Immediately I want to leave, but I picture their conversation halting, them all asking what had upset me, and saying patronising shit like, 'We're only *messing*'. Or worse, the whole dozen of them laughing as I leave, saying things about being sensitive, about being like a little girl.

'Come on,' I say to Emma a minute later.

'Where you off?' Morgan barks when he sees us get up.

I make the "off for another drink" motion, jiggling my hand in front of my mouth.

'Mine's a beer. Cheers and thanks.'

No one else seems to notice us go.

'What's up?' Emma asks on the end of my hand as I lead her through the bar.

'I don't want to be here anymore. Everyone's pissed and it's doing my head in.'

'Don't you want a drink?'

'Not really.'

We walk back, having barely been out five minutes. We watch *QI* in the living room for an hour and drink tea, have sex on the floor of my bedroom. Sometime after ten we're lying in bed, Emma half-asleep on my chest, when Ant rings to see where I went and what was wrong with me.

'Just wasn't my thing tonight,' I say.

He sounds to be outside a pub.

'Was it what I said?'

'Well, it just wasn't. You know.' I do a big sigh.

'You know I was just playing.'

'It wasn't like you normally are. It wasn't the same.'

Neither of us say anything. I hang up.

54

I wash my hands. Wash my hands. Try to stab the toilet door's lock open with the end of my wet finger. Four attempts and it doesn't work. I'm touching it too much; it's defeating the purpose. I get it on the fifth, but my knuckle catches the door handle, and the edge of the lock goes slightly under my fingernail. I turn back and wash my hands again. Then once more. Go into the kitchen and dry them on some paper towel.

Mum comes through the back door carrying a little stack of plant pots and a window-cleaning spray.

'Can you please shift these shoes, Christopher?' she says, kicking one out of her way as she goes through to the garage.

The litter of shoes by the door. Pairs of Dad's, Jordan's, even Mum's. I watch them for a moment, angry that she'd make me do this after I've just got my hands clean. I push one pair together with a foot, then through my sock slide the walls of both shoes between my big toe and second toe. I scrunch my foot to make a kind of fist. It holds the shoes well enough to drag them along the lino whilst I hop back with the other foot.

'For God's sake,' Mum says, emerging from the hall. 'Move.'

She picks all the shoes up in her arms, takes them through to the garage and throws them in. Comes back, snatches the last pair from my toes.

'What?' I say.

'Well what the hell are you trying to be? A flamingo? You can't be so bloody precious.' She puts a hand on the back of a kitchen chair. I must remember not to touch where her hand is now. 'You get dirty, Chris. You can't avoid it. So long as you wash your hands before you eat and after the loo. Look at the state of yours. They're bleeding.'

Then don't make me wash them again.

I go into the garage and put the shoes on the rack with my fingers.

If I wash my hands now, is it worse? I've got open wounds. As I lather the soap and water, the shoe germs on my fingertips will mix in and enter the cracks. Direct to the bloodstream.

'What you doing?' Jordan says in the doorway, catching me stood in the semi-dark staring at nothing.

'Sorting shoes.'

Mum's turning soil in the garden. Bentley's lying beside her. When he sees me slot my feet into the flip-flops I keep by the back door and head down the garden, he gets to his feet and mounts the football. His tail flickers with his high-speed humping. Then he slumps off it, eyes wide and belly throbbing, as though shocked at what he's done.

'You alright, then?' Mum asks, squatted down on the edge of the grass with an old pair of Marigolds on, stabbing away at the mud.

'Yeah.'

I don't dare say what I want to. Don't know how to word it. Even though I've laid the groundwork.

She looks up and squints, her face in a mottled flush. 'What's up?'

'I just don't know what to do about Devon. I don't know what you expect me to do. I've told you I can't do it.'

Mum starts digging again. I stand and wait. Bentley runs round the ball, his cheek never parting contact with it.

'I think you'll do it. You've managed college. You've managed your exams, now.'

'It's not the same, Mum. It's worse. Much worse. It's impossible. You don't *get* how – how it's impossible.'

The little fork jabs and twists the soil until it's fluffy and darker. A big chod of clay's unearthed; she hits it with the edge of the fork until it splits down the middle. 'James was struggling, wasn't he? I can remember our first time to Florida when he had that...' she finds the right words, whilst I recall looking out the rented car's windows, up at the neon signs in the dark above us, lost in America, Dad pulling into the car park of a fast food place and James sprinting inside '...that sort of panic going on. But then he went on that holiday to Spain. And he was extremely nervous about going. He almost cancelled on them. He mentioned it a few times. But he pulled himself together and went, not that I was *overly* pleased about him going. And he was fine.'

'I'm not the same as him,' I say. 'You keep saying about Spain but we're different. I can't just pull myself together. If James had this thing I've got, it was only for a little while. Mine won't just go. This could make it worse.'

'But if you don't come, you'll never know. And think what you might be gaining.'

'Mum, I'm not going. The sooner you get it the better. You need to understand now, so you're not all leaving the house on the morning a few weeks from now and shocked when I say I'm not coming.'

Her "okay" is small.

55

I punch the bag: jab-jab-haymaker. The chains rattle. I skip round as it swings, catch it when it's up. Punch after punch. Dark patches of blood on its blue skin dotted like stamps, spreading, joining each other.

56

'How the hell does Elliot do this all his life?' I ask Dad one lunchtime. 'Just making windows, making windows. Forever.'

'Get your arse through uni and you won't have to do this kind of work,' Dad says. 'But for the lads, it's just life. Sometimes that's all there is.'

I try to wolf my dinner before Dad finishes his and starts picking his nose. If I'm lucky, he'll put *House* on, where genius doctors chase down an elusive illness that threatens to kill a patient. But we only have time to see quarter of an hour before returning to the workshop; we'll leave just when they think they've cured the patient, before he or she starts fitting like crazy and all bets are off again.

Every day at work I think about Devon. Whether my family will leave me behind without another fight. It's only two weeks and six days away. Why am I nervous if I've resolved not to go?

57

'Aren't you having yours?' Dad says, divvying his portion of curry from the foil takeaway trays. Breaking a poppadum up and tucking it into the rice on the side of his plate.

It smells so fucking good.

'I'll have it later on.'

'Chris won't have Surma before he's back from Emma's,' Mum says.

Actually it's not until I've been to Emma's tonight, *and* had my driving lesson tomorrow morning. Then it'll be Surma o'clock.

'Are you afraid it'll tickle your stomach?' he says, then literally swoops in to tickle me with his free hand on his way through to the living room.

I laugh and wish I was like him. It's a Thursday evening; he's driving to Wales at the crack of dawn tomorrow.

Whilst they eat I put *Halo 3* on upstairs, though I can't decide which campaign mission to play: each one is linked to last autumn. Coming home from the cold loops around Barton, my fingers too seized-up to play.

'You fit?' Dad shouts up the stairs.

'Yeah.'

Does he know I'm not coming to Devon? Has Mum told him? There's no way he'd be so nice if he knew. He'd go back to that tired voice, hardly looking at me at all. I don't know if I can be the one to tell him.

Broad daylight at half seven. It's a watery daylight, I think, glancing at the crisscross of vapour trail scars in the apricot sky, before I duck into Dad's BMW. Only this time of year has it, when the sun makes its long, long descent from the very top of the sky. I don't feel wholly awake.

We pass the picnic island's concrete tables where no one ever eats and the slowly crumbling lone house where that old man was murdered.

'Your mother tells me you're thinking of not coming to Devon.'

I brace myself.

'That's nonsense,' he says. 'You're coming. I know it's hard for you. I know it's very hard for you. And I know I don't get it. But whatever you're afraid of doesn't matter. You're with your family, who love you. Okay?'

It knocks the wind out of me. It's one of the strangest things I've ever heard him say.

'Okay,' I say.

It's a lie, and I prepare to notice the lie's wrongness, the retribution it promises, nestle in the back of my skull, a feeling I can only describe as citrusy. But it doesn't come.

Dad's never said he loves me. I've never said it to him. Nor to any of my family. None of us have ever, in my life, mentioned loving each other. That's not to say we don't. It goes unspoken.

'Let's have a tea, Lis,' Emma's dad says.

Emma's mum pushes away the plastic TV dinner table with her laptop on and gets up from the sofa. On her way to the kitchen she asks Emma's older brother and sister, Eric and Miranda, if they want one, then Emma, then me.

'Yeah, go on then, please,' I say.

She stops halfway out the door and reverses back in. 'What? Am I hearing things?'

'Are you feeling alright, Chris?' Emma's dad says.

I sure hope so.

Emma, lounging with her legs hung over mine, tugs my t-shirt and goes, 'Ooh!'

Eric's sat against the wall, scratching their new dog Dot and watching TV. He notices the tray of buns his mum's brought in and reaches up for one.

Miranda scoffs, 'Aren't you going to wash your hands? They're fucking filthy.'

'Fuck off, are they,' he says.

'They are black, honey,' Emma's mum says from the kitchen.

'What is it, that black stuff?' Miranda asks.

'I was helping plough the Coopers', wasn't I?'

'With your hands?'

'Jesus!' Eric licks his hands, scrubs them on the carpet and gets a bun.

When I head out to the square to meet Dad, he gets out his car and goes round to the passenger side, leaving the driver's door open. I try not to grin. As I climb in, the car roars; I don't know what's going on and Dad's slapping my leg. Turns out I've trodden on the accelerator.

'Smoothly does it,' I say.[64]

Driving it feels as easy as if I was playing Xbox. On the long straight into New Holland I put my foot down; the pedal hits the floor and then clicks down a little notch further. The car drops down a few gears and the revs shoot up; it's fast enough to feel that sensation of being pinned into my seat.

'Steady on, then,' Dad laughs when he sees we're nearing 130mph.

58

Squeeze the crisp packets to see if they are sealed. Maybe a sniff, too. Check the best before date. If the date is printed in numbers, are you sure the day and month are the British way round? If it's the American way round, that means it's out of date. Is this food brand likely to be from America?

---

[64] Even if my own hands don't show it, in my head I'm hesitating before touching the steering wheel. But fuck it, they're already filthy. And there's another two weeks and a day until Devon; that's time enough to get ill and recover, right?

I'm always tasting consciously, tasting hard. Abandoning what I eat if there's an irregularity in taste or texture. But I know a waste of food must be sinful, since there are others in this world who starve. So one option means poisoning and the other means punishment. My food often goes cold[65] whilst I sit deliberating; people ask why I'm not moving. I'm trying to make sense. Internally asking for a sign.

I open the fridge by hooking my foot under its door, since Dad regularly comes through from the living room after a nose-picking session to open the fridge by its wooden knob for a snack. I take a yoghurt and check the seal hasn't been broken, lift the edge flaps of the lid, check for residue of other yoghurts from the factory, dents in the plastic. Is it airtight? I give it a squeeze[66], a firmer second squeeze[67], a third – it pops.[68] Globs dot everywhere. I scrub all the surfaces so future food isn't prepared where the yoghurt specks landed. Then I scrub the surfaces where I *can't* see yoghurt specks.

59

Mum uses a sachet of descaler to clear the clumps of limescale our hard water deposits in the kettle. The sharp smell ignites a memory of being five, peeling yellowed sellotape off a cupboard side and smelling its sticky face.

'Are you sure it's okay to drink now?' I say, three hours later.

'I've boiled and re-boiled the kettle. Emptied it each time, like the sachet says. I've even done it a third time. And swilled it out

---

[65] And aren't there more germs in food that's been left to go cold? So I should leave it. But to leave it is a waste, which is a sin.

[66] Did I squeeze hard enough to know?

[67] Did the pot just give a little? Is it a bit deflated compared to the first squeeze? Is there a tiny gap where air can *just* pass through, enough for this yoghurt to have gone bad? I can't fucking tell!

[68] Now I *have* to eat it to avoid punishment.

God knows how much. Your dad and I have had a drink, since. Drink your bloody tea.'

I lift the cup to my nose and smell the steam for traces of descaler.[69]

'Anyway, you know what day it is tomorrow, don't you?' Mum says.

I frown at her for a moment, then beam like I'm seven again and it's Christmas.

'Longest day?'

Mum grins and rubs her hands together, her shoulders hunched up to her ears.

'Oooh!' I put my cup down and hug her, putting on an old man's voice. 'The nights'll be pulling in soon.'

She laughs. Mum hates the dark nights as much as the next English person, but seems to find my joy in it endearing enough to have counted down to this longest day with me.

And now we're over the crest. Time for the long downhill into winter.

60

I wash the rubber buds of my earphones in watered-down Domestos. Using earphones over time must make them swarm

---

[69] I may wish Mum hadn't used this chemical cleaner today, when Emma's coming round later, and ingesting a trace of it might lead to poisoning, but leaving the kettle alone might have been just as bad. Are the sediments in hard water harmful? Remember when James held up a freshly poured glass of cold water that time, and showed me the white bits swirling round the bottom like a snow globe?

with bacteria.[70] My ears might get an infection, and this infection might work into my head, down the tubes into my nose, my oesophagus, my stomach.[71]

Then I wash my hands a few times. Go into my parents' en suite and run my finger through Mum's tub of hand moisturiser, but hesitate just as I'm about to apply it to my cracked knuckles. What if Mum's been in contact with an ill person within the lifetime of this tub, then touched this moisturiser, which incubated the germs like the agar jelly in petri dishes we used to study in Biology class, and I'm about to apply it to broken skin, almost directly into the bloodstream? I wipe it off my finger with tissue, flush it down the toilet with my foot, wash my hands. But this is all in my parents' en suite. It makes me uncomfortable to be in here: last summer, I used this toilet just as Emma arrived, and was nervous the whole time she was here. That day, that *state*, haunts the taps, the carpet, the towels, the lead-patterned glass. So I go through to the main bathroom, holding out my dripping hands[72], and wash them another two times in that sink. Take my socks off with my feet and put them in the wash basket.[73]

---

[70] So said Holly, who in Year Nine turned round from her bench in Science class to check out Lex's iPod Mini. 'And the way earphones shut-in your ears, and that tiny bit of vibration from the inner speaker: it makes you produce wax quicker,' she said, whilst my eyes focused on the wisps of hair above her lip and around her cheeks.

[71] I think about that episode of *The Simpsons* when Principal Skinner opens the box of what he thinks is a new juicer, but a plague of cartoon germs swarm out. "Good Lord," he shouts, "flu germs entering every orifice in my head!"

[72] But where does this dirty water land? My clothes? The carpet, which will transfer onto me another time? Or transfer onto my parents or Jordan, who will subsequently get ill, which will then pass on to me? I'm positive I felt a drop of it hit my toe.

[73] The lid of the wash basket is where folded towels are often laid. Some people, including me in the past, use a fresh towel and think, *well it's hardly used*. So they re-fold it and put it back on the wash basket lid. That means over the years, countless *used towels* of varying degrees have been on this lid. That's why I only use towels straight out the airing cupboard, that haven't touched this lid. And that's why, after lifting the lid up now to put my socks in, I wash my hands again. Then again.

61

James stays at uni as long as possible, until the day they have to leave halls. He arrives home in Granddad's old Fiesta, Dad following behind. I go out to meet them; our brick drive is warm under my socks.

The cars are stuffed. We unload guitars and amps, a little coffee table, a swivel chair, clothes, bin bags of washing, rattling boxes. As we stack it all in the garage, there's a hopeful permanence to it: he must be staying a while.

He comes to work at Dad's. One dinner we walk to the chippy, and on our way back find a shortcut path that runs behind the industrial estate; big, noisy trees with spinning leaves hang over us, and the sun must be as high as it'll ever be. James says this doesn't feel like home anymore.

Dad takes me out to practise driving in Mum's Fiesta whenever we get the chance. Out in the sticks behind Goxhill, I swing us round a blind corner; an oncoming combine harvester, only metres away, swerves a little but doesn't have the space to let us past. Dad says 'Jesus!' and I bump the car up the verge to avoid colliding with, or getting crushed under, those gigantic wheels. Later on when I'm telling the story to Emma, it strikes me that the whole experience didn't make me feel anything.

I pray to God whenever I remember. Ask him to look over my family and Emma. Then I go on to wider appeals: war veterans, the third world.

My feet itch at night.

'You alright?' James says, turning away from the screen to see me standing in the door.

He's sat at the head of my bed, with the pillow against the wall to rest his back on, playing PS3. The bed covers have to be changed now, which Mum only did yesterday; she'll be on to me. Fuck's sake.

'Yeah.' I come in and sit at the desk chair. Try to watch him play and forget about his arse sitting right where I rest my head at night.[74] But I can't. 'Just get up a sec.'

'Why?'

'Just do it.' I swipe my hand, gesturing him to move.

He pauses the game and gets off the bed. I pull the covers up the wall, over the pillow.

'Okay,' I say.

The lesser of two evils. The way my room's assembled makes it difficult to sit here on the chair and still see the TV, so it's got to be the bed, really. Why didn't I think of this, last time I arranged the room?

James sits back down. 'What's that in aid of?'

I'm immediately wound up whenever I find him in here. He tries talking to me but my answers are short. It might be because he was sick December before last, and I still worry there's a modicum of it left for me to catch. Maybe it's because he often scratches his crotch. There's just an unhealthy aura about him. He's underweight, delicate. He looks unhappy. Then I realise what I'm thinking, how I'm being: it's terrible. It's unforgiveable.

So I say, 'Don't you think it's broken that the pistols seem to do more damage than the assault rifles?' and try to let it go that James is holding the PS3 controller.

'It's the enemies ducking and diving. They take so much damage.'

He's playing through *Uncharted*. He reaches a point where you get to man a massive machine gun and mow down a wave of bad guys. I can't play this bit anymore. Even in the light-hearted presentation of *Uncharted* – a videogame's answer to *Indiana Jones*, where violence is innocuous, funny, and served with a regular quip – it

---

[74] It's not just that it's his arse there – though that does play a massive part, its germs seeping through his underwear and jeans ('It just came over me out of nowhere!') – it's his jeans. I picture everywhere they've been, in his halls of residence, on other friend's beds and sofas, on the seats at Nottingham Uni, the canteens and lecture theatres, the public transports he's always riding. And every arse that's sat on every seat he's sat on. All congregating into his jeans, and now wiping on the top of my bed.

reminds me of real slaughter: the attack on Normandy, the Somme. I would be punished for playing it.

62

A plume of steam hits my face when I open the dishwasher.[75] I pull the tray out and take a glass that's hot in my hands. James sits at the table, looking down at his phone. Jordan paws a knife and fork out the drawer. Dad says to him, 'At least you've sorted yourself, Jordan. Hey?' Jordan turns on his heel and opens the drawer again. Mum uses one of those big spoons with battlements round the edges to serve spaghetti across five plates. I rinse my glass under the tap, pour it out, fill it up, pour it out. Feel how cold the water is. Fill the glass, pour it out.

Mum stands beside me with a pot, lid and battlement spoon in her hands.

'You're rinsing a glass that's just come out the dishwasher.'

'Yes.'

'Doesn't make sense, Chris.'

'Then don't watch me.'

I spend the afternoon rearranging my room. I wash my hands after touching a dusty lamp wire and a fifty pence recovered from behind some drawers, after rifling through a few of James's old clothes left in the cupboard[76], after moving the wicker chair and its unwashed clothes with stories to tell, after touching the underside of my bed to pull it and the naked frame beneath the valance when I push it.

---

[75] Is dishwasher steam harmful? Does it contain the bacteria of the formerly dirty – and surely not *completely* clean now – dishes? Is all that shit now on my face? I mustn't lick my lips or sniff too hard.

[76] All year, I've kept James's left-behind clothes to the right of the cupboard and used an old jacket I won't wear anymore as a partition to keep them from touching my clothes on the left.

After every use of the hoover, when hulking the furniture uncovers a greyed patch of carpet. After touching a duster. Or the handle of the Drawer of Sin, which at one point trundles open[77] whilst I'm dragging it and touches my shin, so I change my jeans. After touching any item that links to my sickness period. After removing the bin bag and placing it into a bigger carrier bag, even though I take the time to do this entirely with my toes.[78]

The carpet itself must have so many invisible sex juices dried into it by now. I try to picture where these are, given that the spots me and Emma have sex in have shifted each time I've rearranged the room. I must be careful not to let belongings touch the carpet. And maybe watch where I tread. And be careful what objects I lay on the bed whilst I polish the tops of drawers. Dirty objects that touch the sheets will dirty my bed, whilst clean objects that touch the parts of the sheets where we've sat and had sex will dirty the objects.

I don't know where to put things anymore. Like this old corkboard that's collected cards handwritten and drawn by hand over the years. I can't arrange it in such a way that all cards, drawings and photos are completely visible. To have one overlap the other

---

[77] Has the signet ring fallen into the Johnny grease?! No. Thank God. Sorry. It was never meant to be back there. I never took notice that it was still there whilst the drawer slowly accumulated its slippery film, and its new purpose. Now the ring's trapped because I no longer dare reach over the grease to get it. And I feel guilty that the only possession I own of my dead grandfather is in such a terrible place. But it's safe, on top of the wooden box. It's not touching the juices. Even in the cloudy excitement of being turned on, if I roll over to grab what we need out this drawer, I open it gently, because opening it too fast will make the ring topple forward into the Sin.

[78] I don't keep anything too dirty in it – more used condoms, wrapped tight in tissue, hid amongst scrunched up paper – but I still find the little wire mesh bin frightening. Radioactive. I don't like standing above it. I don't like it being near things that I touch. Even sat there to the right of the trolley I keep games consoles on, I wonder whether its pollution will settle onto the trolley's handle and flat surfaces like warm breath onto a cold mirror. And is it even my bin? It's identical to James's, and I can't remember if, when I moved into this room last year, I brought my bin in and swapped them round or not. If it's James's ex bin, what did *he* put in it over the years? When the bin bag's removed, it reveals faint brownish marks on the bottom like dried tea. I think about the bin a lot.

means I value one person, or one person's efforts, over another. And something tells me that's punishable.

Below the Drawer of Sin is a drawer chock-full of bits and bobs, and I can't part with one item. Not the old scart-to-aerial adapter we used in the 90s for our N64, the rechargeable batteries that can't be charged anymore, some Olympic logo badge that snuck in there, a handful of empty metal lighters I've collected since I was young enough for them to be serious contraband, a slack handful of those beaded surfer necklaces you buy on holidays, a lime-green Gameboy Colour, the clay ashtray I made next to Ant in Year Eleven Art class that now holds dozens of Emma's hair grips, a wad of cards and instruction booklets. I pick these things up to throw away but feel there's an importance to them that I don't understand. They must stay in here.

Evening comes, and I feel a promise of punishment settle into my timeline and take root. The liquid voice of 'Hayling' by FC Kahuna plays on my stereo, telling me, "don't think about all those things you fear". I want its message to sink into me.

I pace my room, looking for more quick changes to make in its layout, then I sit on the edge of my bed and hold my face. My windows are thrown wide open but no air comes in. I don't feel well. Emma's about to arrive and I don't want her to.

63

The light goes green. The Citroen is easy to stall. Its tiny clutch pedal depresses no deeper than a button. I bring it up carefully as possible whilst applying revs, releasing the hand brake. We roll backwards. I slam the foot brake. Pull up the hand brake. Try again. Engine roars. Car rolls backwards. By my third attempt, the light's cycled back to red. I forgot to put the car in gear. This must be a fail. When I finally get going, I see the examiner do a little tick or scribble on his board. It's okay. It might just be a minor.

'*What* colour is that red light?' the examiner shouts, stamping his pedals and stopping the car so hard my seatbelt clicks still and I feel the tyres skid.

'Red,' I say. That's that then.

'What you fucking done?' my driving instructor says back at the centre when I get out the car and shake my head. I can't help but smile a bit, despite being so pissed at myself. Missing a red light.

Maybe because I kept clear of sinful things for days leading up to this, I wasn't nervous this morning. But I am now. I hoped I could pass this test and beg Mum to let me drive her Fiesta down to Devon if I paid for fuel. It would've saved me. I'll be stuck in Dad's car now, going where my family goes.

At home I put *Grand Theft Auto* on. James comes in and puts a tea down beside me. 'Sorry about the test, man,' he says. Using "man" is new; he's picked it up from Nottingham.

'Cheers,' I say, slightly uplifted from a deep sulk.

On the game, my car hurtles through the traffic in Liberty City. But it catches the rear bumper of the car in front, which pings me off the road. I mow down the pedestrians on the sidewalk. They bounce off my car, roll over the top of it. The bonnet's covered in blood. I plough through cones and barriers and rock over some roadworks, back onto the road, not before a guy with a hardhat and fluorescent bib goes under my wheels. The police catch wind and strike up their sirens.

'Reminiscent of how my driving test went down,' I grumble.

James starts laughing.

'Come on,' he says. And I start laughing too.

64

'You been in a fight?' Foxy says.

'Eh?' Then I remember, and inspect my knuckles as though their state is quite new. 'No, these are, like, from – I caught them at work reaching under something.'

Normally they'd be hidden, but I haven't worn lifting gloves in ages: they get full of sweat. They stink over time. Not the kind of material I want rubbing against the torn skin on the back of my knuckles. Even my own germs are still germs.

When I grab the curling bar, I feel the sting of my knuckles opening, and as I curl the bar up to my chest, see the spots of blood.

65

'Isn't James awake?' I ask Dad in the kitchen before work, pouring Crunchy Nut into a bowl. Even as I ask, I prepare myself to hear Dad say he's ill. He's sick. He's got diarrhoea.

And as though I'm psychic, Dad says, 'He's not coming in. He said he isn't well.'

In the minute space between each word of his answer, I fill out the rest, and recall every breathing-distance interaction I've had with James in the last few days, what he's touched of mine, what I've touched of his. Devon is only four nights away.

What the fuck's wrong with James?

'What's up with him?'

'Dunno.' Dad takes his tea through to the lounge.

More people work at Humber Windows. Fitters stand outside by the shutters in the cool morning; they smoke and discuss their day, pointing up at the doors and down at the "trim" laid across the floor. Dad charges about whistling 'Rudebox' through his teeth. He tells me about who's "on the books" and who's a "subby". What work contract looks promising, what's slipped through his fingers. He leans back on his desk chair, goes '*Pfff*!' and laughs. 'It's madness.' Deliveries arrive all day. The bloke who now runs Bright-Spec drops off enquiries he's secretly paying Dad to price up and draw.

We go home at lunch and make a corned beef sandwich and catch twenty minutes of *House*. James is in the kitchen making food as we clear our plates and I shove my feet into my old trainers. 'What's the matter, then?' Dad asks him.

'Headache. Diarrhoea,' James says, cutting a sandwich, sucking chutney off the knife and chucking it in the sink. The second word is like fire alarms blaring from every wall. In a furious overdrive, I'm looking at everything he's touching, from the breadboard to the bread bag, the knife, the sink it's clattered into, the fridge, butter, where he's stood, in case feet can transmit the illness. Everything he's touched all day, the last few days, those thousands of items, surfaces, machine-gunning through my mind. Things I can't touch now. I need to get out. I'm breathing the same air from the lungs he's sighed from whilst sitting on the toilet squirting shit into the water. How well did he wash his hands? Which bathrooms has he used? Atoms, atoms.

'Very good,' Dad says, smacking James on the back. 'Come on,' he says to me. Now I think about that hand Dad just touched him with.

I work with Elliot's stepson Greg on the plastic windows whilst Elliot does the complicated projects, quiet and seemingly happy. All afternoon I'm thinking about surfaces, bacteria, diarrhoea, the long drive to Devon, the long walks over Dartmoor, my stomach cramping, absolutely desperate for a shit, begging my Dad to pull over and running up the motorway bank for somewhere to squat, or not making it at all and shitting right there in the car despite my terrified effort to keep it in, the tangible smell, my family's reactions, their expressive eyes, how it will anchor in their memories, their perspective of me. This is what will happen. It's been decided. We're leaving on Saturday: I'll just have time to catch it by then.

After work I wait in Dad's office whilst another bloke from Bright-Spec comes in to ask for a job. He says the Hobarts have been telling their ex-employees that they paid Dad a year's salary as a farewell gift when he left. Dad starts laughing.

I get home and go upstairs to change my clothes. **James is sat on my chair playing the PS3.**

I don't fucking believe it.

The room is stuffy, fucking *full* with the airborne germs. This is where I've got to sleep and spend the night gradually inhaling those particles, like a pond filter supping algae, until I contain it all. Is he *trying* to pass it on? How could you go in someone else's room when you're ill? How could you touch their stuff? My controller, my TV remote, my seat, the carpet where he's walked.

'Alright?' James turns his head a bit whilst his eyes stay fixed to the screen.

I get changed without breathing and leave before I see any more.
'Headache. Diarrhoea.'

Like it's nothing. Like it won't spread.

The bottle says it kills 99.9% of germs. I spray it onto a square of kitchen roll, hold the PS3 controller with a finger and thumb placed where James was least likely to have touched, start massaging in the cleaner. I take the spray upstairs to go round the other surfaces.

66

Some objects are comforting: the Swiss Army knife Dad bought me one Christmas, my copy of *Lord of the Rings*, my earphones and iPod, and the scratty old backpack I stow these things into on the Friday evening.

The second I've packed, I unzip my bag to check that nothing's missing.

I go to Emma's for a couple of hours.[79] Come home and wash my hands until the water scalds me. Throw my clothes in the wash basket, wash my hands again. Turn the shower on. Take my boxers off, take my socks off with my feet. Bunch it all together between my big and second toe and drop it into the basket. It's sensible to have clean hands before getting into the shower. It's equally sensible

---

[79] If I breathe deeply, dust will go straight into my lungs. If I breathe nice and slow, a good fraction of it should settle around the inside of my nose, which I can clean later with a wet tissue. Brushing a foot over the long carpet, ruffling their new dog's fur or patting a sofa cushion will release more dust into the air. Try to stay still. Breathe slow.

to clean your hands after getting *out* of the shower: you've just been touching your arse, your junk, the moist crevices of your body, even if it's to clean them. So I wash my hands after showering. Then wash them after pulling on my trousers. I check my bag again. Phone and laptop chargers. Batteries for my camera. Emergency tablets in the side pocket: the last Stemetil, Imodium, painkillers. In the opposite side pocket is a small handful of graphite powder spilt from a plastic film canister, a tiny rag stained with ink, a rectangle of mezzotint copper, none of which I can throw away.

Nerves don't keep me up at night. Scenarios of me being ill, and of things being okay, stir together. I send a prayer. I drift asleep.

Whilst my family eat breakfast I check my bag a dozen times, looking between it and my checklist. My suitcase is arranged so that socks don't touch boxers or t-shirts, hair gel and deodorant don't touch boxers, and nothing touches the oxytetracycline. Strictly no shoes or belts. Sandwich bags are useful for dividing the toiletries and tablets. The clothes will no doubt lose their position on the journey, but I still carry the suitcase horizontally down the stairs and lay it carefully into the car's boot. Careful not to let the handle of James's kitbag anywhere near my case.

Wait, hang on. I hoik the case back out, lay it on the drive and open it. The oxytetracycline are *definitely* there. There are enough to last me. I touch the pack. Fold it back into the sandwich bag. Close the case. Run upstairs and check my bag again. Touch the pills in the side pocket. Hold the charging wires between my fingers. Wash my hands a few times.

Dad carries bags through the hall, turning side-on to pass James. 'You fit?' Dad says. 'Still got a runny bottom?'

'Not so bad, now.' James leans his satchel on the wall and puts his feet into his shoes.

He must be beyond contagion now. 'Not so bad.' That's not so bad. But look at him. He grabs his bag and asks if I'm coming. Goes out the door for an eight-hour ride, knowing he might be ill. He truly cured himself of that taste he had of whatever's wrong with me. He did it by himself, without a counsellor. I always wish I was like Jordan: calm no matter where he goes. But maybe I should wish I was like James: calm despite misfortune often buffeting against him. It's like he just accepts that the worst might happen.

Dad comes back in and picks up the box by the door: food Mum's packed for the hut we're staying in. The day of my A Level results is in the middle of the holidays. Dad's offered to drive me all the way up here for the night to get them.

'All set?' he asks.

'Think so.'[80] I walk past him to the front door.

'Good lad.'

Dad sits in the car and waits for everyone to get in. Mum's last, locking up every window, then finally the front door. She slots a map between her seat and the centre armrest.

It's cramped back here. Jordan's leg rests against mine. He's between me and James. Does that mean Jordan will catch James's bug before me? Will he suck up a good quantity of the air James breathes before it reaches me? He opens his Sudoku book and taps a chewed-up pen against his teeth. Dad puts the car in reverse and backs us out the drive.

Fucking hell[81], I'm doing this. We're off.

---

[80] Images, images, images. Vomiting, shitting, vomiting, shitting. In the car, across my family, in my boxers, down onto the floor between my feet, beside the hard shoulder as motorway traffic gushes by, down a ditch, behind a hedge. Will there be hiding places? How much sooner does the sun set now than it did at the end of June? Would my family be kind enough to leave me if we pulled over and I ran away from the car, into the trees? Would they be kind enough to drive on? Have I packed enough of the *good* boxers, that feel restrictive like a diaper? I should check again. Will oxytetracycline save me from eight hours in the car with James's illness-leaden breath? From the food we eat down there? The new surfaces I touch?

[81] Sorry, it just slipped out. Have I cursed the trip? "Slipped out", like shit will when I become ill. No, it's not related. I just said it by accident, out of habit. 'It's back to the routine,' as Dad said. No, not back to how I was. No. Sorry.

Acknowledgements

Martin Goodman convinced me that this was a story worth telling; he's been my supervisor and friend from start to end. Kate Galvin and Judith Dyson warmly introduced me to their wonderful department. Robyn, Kirndeep, Jordan, Eve and Paula blazed through early drafts; Jonathan and Peter examined later drafts. Matt helped tease out those shyer memories. My parents have tirelessly supported me year after year, even whilst knowing that for all their efforts, their reward would be a book that hurts to read.

Printed in the USA
CPSIA information can be obtained
at www.ICGtesting.com
JSHW011027010424
60342JS00006B/7